Erasing Pain

Erasing Pain

New Treatments

from the World-Famous

Rusk Institute's Medical Specialists

Mathew H. M. Lee, M.D.
Medical Director, Rusk Institute

and

Mary F. Bezkor, M.D.
Physical Medicine and Rehabilitation, Rusk Institute

Thomas Dunne Books
St. Martin's Griffin ⚘ New York

THOMAS DUNNE BOOKS.
An imprint of St. Martin's Press.

www.stmartins.com

Book design by Richard Oriolo

Library of Congress Cataloging-in-Publication Data

Lee, Mathew H. M.
    Erasing pain : new treatments from the world-famous Rusk Institute's medical
specialists / by Mathew H. M. Lee and Mary F. Bezkor.
        p. cm.
    Includes index.
    ISBN 0-312-24228-X (hc)
    ISBN 0-312-30265-7 (pbk)
    1. Pain—Treatment. I. Bezkor, Mary F. II. Howard A. Rusk Institute of
Rehabilitation Medicine. III. Title.

RB127.L38 2001
616'.0472—dc21   2001041896

First St. Martin's Griffin Edition: September 2002

10 9 8 7 6 5 4 3 2 1

This book is dedicated to our courageous patients who suffer, and through them we learn and share the best therapeutic approaches.

Contents

Acknowledgments

We are grateful to Lois Smith, Izumi Cabrera, and Linda Moy for their gracious help in the tedious manuscript preparations and revisions; to George Walsh for his editorial and research expertise; and to the publishing staff of Thomas Dunne Books.

Part One

What We Do at the Rusk Institute

What is the Rusk Institute, and how did it evolve?

Just after World War II, the pioneering Howard A. Rusk, M.D., recognizing the need for a special type of medical facility, one that would use a team approach to treating illnesses and relieving pain, founded the Rusk Institute of Rehabilitation Medicine in New York City. It was the world's first such facility to treat the entire patient, addressing emotional, psychological, and social needs as well as ailments and disabilities. Over the years, hundreds of thousands of sufferers have benefited from its comprehensive programs; today, operating under the umbrella of the New York University Medical Center, it is the largest such university-affiliated institute in the country.

How is the treatment organized?

Each patient is cared for individually, by a specially created rehabilitation team. The physiatrist (a physician specializing in rehabilitation medicine) acts as the group's leader, designing overall care and directing its implementation.

All physiatrists at Rusk, who maintain their private practices, are faculty members of the NYU School of Medicine's Department of Rehabilitation Medicine. Team members under their supervision are expert in such fields as physical therapy, occupational therapy, nursing, speech pathology, vocational rehabilitation, psychology, prosthetics and orthotics, and horticultural and music therapy.

Why are you writing this book?

We believe that the medical profession often treats patient pain inadequately, sometimes badly. Most doctors are poorly trained in how to deal with the phenomenon, and sufferers are becoming more and more impatient with their lot. As proof, witness the national controversy over the role of pain in justifying the legalization of marijuana and even assisted suicide.

For decades Rusk has been the world's most prestigious pain-management clinic. But untold numbers of sufferers will never see the inside of our facility. Now, in this concise question-and-answer book, we hope to inform these people about our clinic and its methods and show them hope that pain can be conquered, or at least alleviated. Our purpose is twofold: to educate patients and to help them communicate more effectively with their own doctors.

One of us, Mathew H. M. Lee, M.D., internationally known in the pain-management community for more than thirty years, is Rusk's longtime medical director. The other, Mary F. Bezkor, M.D., is a senior Rusk specialist in physical medicine. Backing us up are Institute colleagues in every discipline who have reviewed and approved our work.

Understand, however, that this book does not pretend to be encyclopedic. Its aim is to teach the medical basics so that patients can ask the questions that lead to informed decisions.

What kind of patients come to Rusk, and how do you help them?

Consider these prototypes:

- Ellen G., a marketing manager in her early fifties, has had lower back pain for years. The operative cause is a slightly bulging disc. Until recently she had been able to control the condition with mild medication. But now the pain is much more intense. Will surgery be necessary? Ellen's X-ray history shows that the condition of the disc has not worsened. Many doctors might suggest surgery anyway. But the Rusk Institute treats the whole patient. We conduct tests, ask questions, search for answers. We note swelling in Ellen's legs and ankles, the result of a sporadic and apparently unrelated circulatory ailment. Questioning reveals that the drug being used to treat the edema is no longer potent. Ellen has kept it in her medicine cabinet too long. The swelling is causing poor posture, both sitting and standing, putting intolerable strain on the disc. We update her edema prescription, teach her good posture, design a stretching program to relax her back muscles. No surgery for Ellen.

- Charles H., forty-five, is a hard-charging homebuilder who owns his own contracting firm. An aging baby boomer, he finds it difficult to realize that he is growing older, that his body cannot take the punishment it did when he was younger. He comes to us with chronic shoulder, elbow, and wrist pains. Developing his patient profile, we learn that Charles jogs daily—accompanied, on a leash, by his equally hard-charging Irish wolfhound. The dog stands thirty inches high and weighs 130 pounds. We gently suggest behavior modification: namely, jogging without the wolfhound. The patient reluctantly agrees. Three months later, no more pain.

- Helen B., a thirty-three-year-old retailer diagnosed with breast cancer, has undergone a successful lumpectomy. Now, weeks later, she is increasingly despondent because of postsurgical pain. Breast tissue surrounding the tumor has been damaged during its removal. Some doctors might simply prescribe pain-killing drugs. But we feel that Helen needs more than medication. We help her structure an overall pain-alleviating plan, one that enables her to control her symptoms. Besides analgesics, its components include exercises, music therapy, positive mental imagery. Soon the pain recedes.

What are the patient's options when seeking pain relief?
The broad categories are medications, surgery, and nonsurgical procedures:

- Medications include analgesics, anti-inflammatory drugs, narcotics, and relaxants and tranquilizers.

- Surgery may call for disc removal or fusion, widening the openings of nerve endings, or bathing an area internally with narcotics.

- Nonsurgical procedures encompass (1) physical agents like deep or superficial heat, cryotherapy (used to reduce swelling), exercise, transcutaneous electrical nerve stimulation (TENS), ultrasound, acupressure, and acupuncture; (2) coping strategies, like behavior modification, biofeedback, and hypnosis; and (3) environmental modification, like changes in what one wears and how one's home or office is furnished.

Pain treatments are continually evolving and broadening, and patients must make themselves knowledgeable about them. They should know, for instance, that thermography often succeeds in pinpointing areas of chronic pain where X rays fail, finding the trouble spots because—owing to impaired circulation—they emit less heat.

How extensive are Rusk's facilities?

Because of its ties to the NYU Medical Center, which has a 726-bed acute-care facility, Rusk provides patients, both adults and children, with an optimal rehabilitation setting, both on an inpatient and outpatient basis. Among the conditions for which we offer remedial programs are aphasia (loss of the ability to articulate or comprehend because of brain damage), amputation, back pain, cardiac problems, cerebral palsy, dysphagia (speech impairment), hand disabilities, head injuries, hip and lower extremity fractures, joint replacements, multiple sclerosis, neuromuscular diseases, Parkinson's disease, pulmonary diseases (asthma, bronchitis, and emphysema), scoliosis (abnormal curvature of the spine), spina bifida (congenital spinal defects), spinal cord injury, sports injuries, stroke, swallowing disorders, traumatic injuries, and vestibular (balance) disorders.

Can you be more specific about your inpatient programs?

Here are a few:

- **Stroke.** Rusk admits some 300 new stroke patients annually, enabling it to develop and maintain a high level of expertise in the most innovative interdisciplinary care, including speech training and psychological consulting.

- **Spinal cord injury (SCI).** Similarly, because Rusk has treated some 1,800 SCI patients over the past fifty years, it can offer the most comprehensive rehabilitation available, including, after discharge, follow-up services.

- **Cerebral palsy.** Since 1986 nearly 400 children with cerebral palsy have experienced significant improvement as a result of our rhizotomy program for reducing spasms.

- **Amputation.** Individuals suffering from limb amputations learn about exercise regimens for strengthening muscle groups, the latest advances in prosthetics, and coping techniques for everyday living.

- **Orthopedics.** This speciality focuses on three areas: joint replacement, orthopedic surgery, and sports injuries, with the rehabilitation team using strength-building therapies to reduce the pain associated with musculoskeletal trauma.

- **Heart disease.** Here our approach to patients with cardiac problems concentrates on reducing stress, minimizing complications, identifying risk, and promoting mobility and exercise.

- **Head trauma.** Brain-injury deficiencies caused by blows, infections, or temporary interruption of the brain's oxygen supply are treated, in part, through cognitive remediation, biofeedback, and horticultural and music therapy.

What should I know about your outpatient programs?

First understand that inpatient therapies often permit sufferers to become outpatients. Take arthritis. Someone in severe arthritic pain can check into Rusk to benefit from the full attention of a rehabilitation team—including exercise through hydrotherapy, splinting, and joint-protection devices.

Then, when the pain becomes manageable, we keep it in remission through outpatient visits. Many other conditions, like the aforementioned heart disease and head trauma, can be treated in the same way.

How are the outpatient programs organized?

Roughly along the following lines, although there is considerable overlap:

- Physical therapy offers individualized exercises to increase strength, endurance, and mobility and is used for such problems as balance disorder, back pain, and hand weakness.

- Occupational therapy is aimed at producing an independent and productive lifestyle and focuses on improving neuromuscular skills, using wheelchairs and prosthetics, and dealing with cognitive deficiencies.

- Speech-language therapy repairs communication functions damaged by illnesses like stroke and head trauma and provides services to children with developmental or acquired disorders.

- Psychological therapy supplies rehabilitative care to sufferers with a wide range of illnesses, from brain tumors to aneurysms, from cancer to stress.

- Cardiac therapy is designed for patients requiring ongoing and comprehensive treatment for problems like angina and the aftermath of angioplasty and bypass surgery.

Is there any illness you don't cover?

Our inpatient and outpatient programs, using both traditional and alternative methods, address the entire spectrum of medical disorders.

Part Two

Questions Patients Ask
Us About Pain

Defining Pain

What is pain?

Pain is any unpleasant sensation. We feel it, with greater or lesser severity, as a result of injury, disease, or emotional disorder. The conduits for pain are nerve endings, or receptors, that are almost everywhere in the body, both externally and internally. When damaged, they reflexively carry the word up the nervous system to the brain, which evaluates the pain and tells us that we are hurting.

Only the person feeling the pain can truly describe it. That is why patients should learn how to communicate with their doctors, who in turn must listen. A common language will then be established. That is the purpose of this book.

What are the common types of pain?

Pain can be acute, when it occurs from a known origin, or chronic, when it has no known origin. Acute pain begins suddenly and ends within a relatively short time. We call pain chronic if it persists for more than six months after the injury or disease or is recurring.

Within these two divisions, sensations can range from sharp or intense to dull or aching. Pain can throb, stab, cut, sear, sting, or feel like pins and needles. Patients should search for the exact words to convey their condition to their doctors.

Some experts believe in a third type of pain: so-called cancer pain, suffered by those with long-term, debilitating illnesses. We disagree. Cancer pain can be defined, more precisely, as a combination of acute and chronic pain.

How does the treatment for acute pain differ from that for chronic pain?

Acute pain, because it has a sudden onset and usually a single cause, is far easier to treat. You identify the cause, remove or alleviate it, and take steps to heal the damage.

Chronic pain, because it is ongoing and may have multiple causes, requires a deeper analysis. The injury should have healed or the disease subsided, but it has not. What other factors are interfering with the healing process? Complicating the equation is the recurrent nature of the pain: The patient, anticipating its coming, can actually reinforce it.

We tell our patients that treating chronic pain requires that we know their lifestyle. Are they overstressed in their career? Are they exercising too much or too little? Are they having personal problems?

To sum up, acute pain can be treated by focusing on the injury or the disease. Chronic pain can be treated only when its multiple causes are identified and the patient realizes that ongoing pain needs ongoing solutions.

What is referred pain?

Pain is said to be "referred" if you feel it in an area of your body that is not actually where the hurt originates. This happens when the nerve endings from different parts of the body share the same neural pathway to the brain. In effect, the brain gets confused. Pain from a heart attack, for instance, may be felt in the arm, neck, or jaws; from a gallbladder attack, in the shoulders.

Because the internal organs are linked from their embryonic beginnings with the skin, which is itself an organ, internal problems often surface far from the source.

What is psychosomatic pain?

We call pain psychosomatic if it originates, in part or in whole, from psychological rather than physical causes. This does not mean that the pain is not real. Some people can easily cope with stressful situations, for example, but others may develop chronic headaches. The patient should not stoically endure, nor the doctor airily dismiss, such miseries.

If you are suffering from psychosomatic pain, you should realize that your brain is responding not just to an immediate cause but to previous experiences. In other words, your brain is being bullied. Treatment requires patient and doctor to recognize the totality of the pressure and then take steps to relieve it.

What happens when the body feels more pain than it can bear?

As pain intensifies, our bodies produce endorphins to help us reduce its impact. These endorphins are hormones that bind with opiates in the brain and thus inhibit unpleasant sensations. But this defense mechanism has its limits.

All individuals have their own pain thresholds, largely depending on their psychological resilience and physical well-being. When that threshold is crossed, the acute-pain sufferer generally loses consciousness; the chronic-pain sufferer falls into depression.

What kinds of pain signal medical emergencies?

Generally speaking, pain signals its urgency if it is unremitting and ever more intense. Some medical emergencies with such signals are cardiac arrests, appendicitis, peptic ulcers, and blood clots.

Can pain be measured?

Everyone's pain is so subjective, so based on individual experience, that it would be foolish to claim we can measure it with total accuracy. We try to turn that subjective weakness into a strength by having patients do the measuring themselves—using a scale of 0 to 10, with 0 being no pain and 10 excruciating pain. The patients keep this record on a daily basis, and more frequently if we think it advisable.

This information is invaluable. Once we see on which days, and at which times of day, individuals' pain peaks, we try to find a connection between the data and the way they lead their lives. Sometimes the solution is simply modifying one's behavior.

Self-measurement provides doctors with a powerful diagnostic tool and engages patients in defining their disorders.

Why is it sometimes so difficult to describe pain?

This usually happens because patients often have no frame of reference for their pain. They are on unfamiliar ground. They become confused—they grope for words. They may feel silly or may be frightened. Their doctors should help them acquire the vocabulary needed to express themselves. Only then can patients properly report their symptoms.

How do the best doctors do this? They take the time to relate to their patients—by listening, by establishing a rapport, by creating a comfort zone. They want to know more than the simple fact that an individual is hurting. They want to know how badly, where, why, and a host of other details.

Why does my doctor seem to underestimate my pain?

Patients know they are in pain. They want their doctors to sympathize. If the doctor does not display the anticipated reaction, the patient thinks he or she does not care or does not have a solution. But the doctor may fully understand and may even be able to help.

There can be any number of reasons for the misunderstanding. As noted, patients may be failing to describe their suffering accurately. Or they may be asking for undue sympathy for what, in reality, is a minor irritant.

Doctors, in turn, may not want to interrupt the patient's story, preferring to listen and learn. Or they may be reserving comment until the results of diagnostic testing are available. Or they may be waiting for enough time to pass to make the patient's own measurement of his or her pain meaningful.

Is it fair to say that pain-management clinics offer patients a multidisciplinary approach to their problems?

Precisely. It's not unusual for a typical pain clinic to offer sufferers a medical team that includes, say, experts in anesthesia, nursing, psychology, physical therapy, and perhaps acupuncture. We at the Rusk Institute fortunately have the resources to push pain management to the limit, taking advantage of the latest developments in the field and drawing on the expertise of hundreds of medical professionals.

What is meant by pain being a "vicious cycle"?

This term applies to people who have chronic, or long-term, pain. You twisted your ankle six months ago, for instance, and it still hurts. The pain is constant, affecting your moods, making you testy and querulous. You take some pills to relieve the pain. But the medication, for one reason or another, is inadequate. Then at night the pain worsens, and insomnia sets in. Finally, because you're not getting enough sleep and because you feel you'll never get better, you fall into depression.

All this time, you've been taking medication: pills for the pain, pills for the insomnia, pills for the depression. You've become a zombie.

The only way out of this "vicious cycle" is to recognize that using medication in this manner is self-defeating. Proper medical care calls for creating a master plan that breaks down the patient's problems, then treats each one separately.

What is the difference between real and imagined pain?

The difficult balance between real and imagined pain may never be solved by the sufferer. It is important for sufferers to communicate their pain and be given affirmation that the experience is believed. At times, the boundaries between real and imagined pain may blur in the treatment process. Diagnostic studies and measurements are of great importance and value. However, for complete recovery, attacking the problem of the internal experience of pain is essential.

Understanding Pain I

How does pain work?

The physiology seems simple, and it all takes place in a split second. Your body receives a stimulus, or sensation, either externally or through an internal organ. The sensation, picked up by a nerve ending, zips up the nervous system and the spinal cord to the brain, which instantly tells you whether the feeling is unpleasant or pleasant. You touch a hot pot on the stove, you drop the pot. Action, reaction.

But the actual workings of the brain, as we now know from PET (position emission tomography) scans, are far more complicated. Different areas of the brain simultaneously focus on the sensation; pose questions like "Have I experienced this pain before?" "Is this the worst it's been?" "Is this the longest-lasting?"; then interpret the data.

The intricacy of this process has pitfalls. With various parts of the brain in effect competing with one another, a surfeit of information can result, causing the patients to become muddled about their condition.

How does the body respond to pain?

Everyone reacts to pain in his or her own way. On the physical level, given the body's complex neurological network, that's understandable.

On the subconscious level, your emotional state affects your response. If you don't like yourself or feel you're friendless or hate your job, you'll be far less likely to take a positive approach to your problem.

Is there "good" pain and "bad" pain?

Of course. Let's say you exercise and work up a sweat. You feel good, but your body aches from the exertion. We call that good pain because you have accomplished something and your body is reacting normally. Or let's say you come home from a day of hunching over a computer. Your neck and shoulders ache from the strain. Your spouse massages the area, gets the circulation going, relaxes the muscles. We call that good pain because you can feel the soreness leaving your body.

Don't forget: Pain is a signal. It's telling you something. The qualifiers *good* and *bad* are just words we're subjectively applying to the process.

Patients should understand this. Let's say you undergo surgery, an invasive procedure. You know you'll feel pain for a brief time afterward, during the recuperative period. But it's good pain because it's a sign that you're healing.

So the term *good pain* is a diagnostic tool. It tells us that the body is working as it's supposed to. What we strive to do is eliminate "bad pain," or at least control it.

Why can't anyone pinpoint the cause of my pain?

Some injuries and illnesses are easier to diagnose than others. When you cut your finger or bump your head, for instance, you know where the pain originates.

Referred pains are another matter. Some are relatively easy to identify, some are not. If a patient has a pain in the chest radiating down the left arm, we suspect the heart may be malfunctioning. Pain beginning around the navel and spreading to the lower right abdomen can mean appendicitis. Pain in the lower back moving up between the shoulder blades may indicate a bad gallbladder. Other cases are more difficult to spot.

Soft-tissue pain around a bone break, for example, is a difficult diagnosis. The bone itself usually has a timetable for healing, depending on which bone it is and the injury's severity. But damage to the soft tissue is different. Diagnosing it, and quantifying the extent of the pain, sometimes involves making an informed guess.

Does pain always signal injury or illness?

Not always. Suppose you twist your knee and go on crutches for a while. The knee heals, but now you feel shoulder pain because of the crutches. That's not an injury, that's soreness coming from little-used muscles. You just have to wait it out.

Other times you may be a victim of your emotions. The memory of pain from an injury in the past comes back to haunt you, triggering pain in the present. Once you understand you're carrying a self-imposed burden, you're taking the first step toward discarding it.

Do some people have a higher tolerance of pain than others, or even feel no pain at all?

Yes. You may have been brought up not to complain and to suffer in silence. But these are just societal attitudes. On a physical level, some people actually have in their genes the capacity to tolerate heavy doses of pain. Perhaps, day in and day out, they produce more endorphins than the rest of us. Individuals who have this unusual trait, which we call congenital absence of pain syndrome, often have a history of repeated injuries.

If you feel no pain at all, of course, you can be in real trouble. People have died from ruptured appendixes, for example, because they do not even know they have a problem.

Pain sends out valuable warnings that help us mitigate bodily injury or stop harmful practices. People with abnormally high pain thresholds are unable to learn from these warnings.

Can the mind make the body more sensitive to pain?

Quite often. If you are anticipating pain, for instance, your worry can intensify the actual pain experience. If you find your surroundings distasteful, your unhappiness can do the same thing.

Your mental and physical states are intertwined. Many people, particularly those in stressful careers, don't eat properly, don't get enough exercise, don't get enough sleep. As a result, they are in chronic low spirits, lowering their resistance to pain. We try to make them see the connection.

Why do severely injured people sometimes feel no pain?

Soldiers on the battlefield, after suffering horrendous injuries, sometimes need no painkillers until they are taken back to a field hospital. The shock of the injury and the relief they feel at still being alive somehow forestall the pain. It's likely that their brains receive a quick, massive dose of endorphins. The individuals do not experience the totality of the pain, and they remain conscious.

Similarly, there are scores of cases of men and even women who somehow find the strength to lift automobiles off children pinned underneath. Not until later do the rescuers feel pain and learn that they have incurred bone fractures from their exertions. System overload produces system shutdown.

Can emotional pain cause physical pain?

Certainly. Emotional trauma, such as that induced by grief and separation, often heightens the body's sensitivity. But sufferers should not separate the psychological from the physical, nor should they feel guilty that their pain may be emotional in origin. Both elements are present, and the pain is not "in their head."

What types of pain do emotions set off?

Your emotional state affects basic bodily functions like blood pressure, heart rate, vascular flow, and gastric acid secretion, causing headaches, irritable bowel syndrome, peptic ulcers, and hypertension.

Are women more likely than men to suffer emotional pain?

We think not. What gives rise to this commonly held belief is that women, because of certain learned-behavior patterns, sometimes exhibit a greater range of emotional responses than men to stress. But, medically speaking, they are not any more likely to be "emotional." Neither a woman's thought processes nor her nervous system is different from a man's.

What are the most common misconceptions about pain?

Some people do not understand that pain, because it is unique for every individual, requires professional treatment. They feel they can deal with their pain by asking someone else how he or she handled a similar problem. They talk to their friends and ask what worked, or didn't work, for them. This leads to many difficulties, particularly with medications. Patients take someone else's pills, and their pain intensifies. They may even die.

Other people believe their pain is a punishment. They feel that they have done something wrong to "deserve" their pain, that it is retribution for past misdeeds. This misconception adds the element of guilt, making it harder to treat the patient.

If a person with guilt feelings has a stroke, for instance, he or she may refuse to undergo rehabilitation, insisting that the stroke is the will of God. We try to reverse this mind-set, stressing to the patient that still being alive means that recovery, not his or her demise, is the will of God.

Does the ability to tolerate pain vary from culture to culture?

Some societies greatly value stoicism. A significant amount of pain must be tolerated before individuals may complain or express their feelings about their pain. This attitude can have grave consequences. Important symptoms may not be detected, because patients keep their own counsel.

On the other extreme, some cultures find it quite acceptable for people to express their feelings about their pain openly and fully, even emphatically. This attitude facilitates venting, which can be helpful. Pain expressed in such an immediate way may help sufferers avoid chronic ailments like ulcers.

Is pain cumulative?

It often can be. Patients cannot help but build up a memory base of the daily and perhaps hourly pains they endure. As time goes on, an individual's anxiety about these sensations may heighten them. Or what begins as an isolated pain may, in the patient's mind, spread throughout the entire body.

Understanding Pain II

Do men and women feel pain differently?

We doubt it. This is not to say that men and women do not anticipate pain differently. In thirty years of acupuncture practice, we can remember only two women who have fainted at the sight of the hair-thin, harmless needles, in contrast to dozens of men. So much for the "weaker sex" stereotype.

Do men and women express their pain in different ways?

Men and women, from culture to culture, may be taught or influenced at an early age to react differently to pain. Even whether a man or woman is communicating with someone of the same or the opposite sex may affect the equation.

Men may feel that they must endure pain, for example, rather than alleviate it. Women may feel less constrained. These societal pressures need to be explored. Patients, before they can be helped, must understand these ingrained patterns.

Similarly, men and women do have some mutually exclusive medical problems—for men, prostatitis; for women, menstrual pain. These gender differences are real, but the pain is equally real—for male and female.

Can men bear some types of pain better than women can, and vice versa?

Only in the sense, we believe, that men commonly are expected to be more stoic than women in dealing with pain. But whether this trait is inculcated or genetic is of little relevance. Patients, regardless of gender, should be encouraged to describe their pain fully.

Do children feel pain differently from adults?

Children feel pain differently because they are usually encountering it for the first time. They have no memory of past suffering and, therefore, no anticipation of future distress. This helps us in treating them, because we can focus on the here and now.

Of course, every experience children have with pain brings them incrementally into the adult sphere. No one looking at the drawings child cancer patients do can fail to recognize their anguish.

Is pain more likely to strike at certain times of day?

It's true that the body's chemistry creates daily biorhythms, or cycles, that contribute to how well you tolerate pain. On top of the cycle, you're likely to ignore, or even forget, your discomfort; on the bottom, you're prone to dwell on it. But if you find your pain worsening each day at a particular time, the cause is usually more prosaic. Perhaps you're sitting too long. Perhaps you're walking too far. Perhaps you're jogging too fast.

Once you associate your activities with your discomfort, you can modify them accordingly. Do you get back pain after sitting thirty minutes at your desk? Get up after twenty minutes to do some stretching. Leg pain after walking a mile? Cut back to half a mile. Knee pain while jogging? Slow down, or remove the pressure on your knees entirely by taking up swimming.

Moderation in all things. It's always good advice.

Why does my pain get worse at night?

During the day you are exposed to all sorts of stimulation: daylight itself, interaction with other people, the details of workplace and household. At night, lacking these stimuli, you're likely to concentrate on your pain, even become obsessed with it. You can ease your discomfort by imagining pleasant images or listening to soothing sounds. Nighttime pain-reduction techniques include guided imagery, calming music, and repetitive prayer.

Do we feel pain while we are asleep?

Sleep, of course, is not uniform. We go from light to deep to rapid-eye-movement, or dream, sleep and back again four or five times a night. But throughout all these stages, our sensory systems are still at work subconsciously.

Let's say you are lying too long on one side, putting too much pressure on an arm or shoulder. Subconsciously you feel the pain; therefore, you turn over. People normally shift position about every fifteen minutes.

In the case of chronic pain, if these subliminal messages are strong enough, they will awaken the sleeper.

Why don't I feel pain until a second or two after an injury?

The initial shock of the injury probably produces a signal delay for a brief moment, which delays the sensory experience. You see the injury, but need an instant to feel it.

Why does rubbing an injured area often ease the discomfort?

Rubbing or massaging an area is a way of confusing the pain signal. Particularly when done with such stimulating agents as alcohol, menthol, and camphor, it becomes a counterirritant, masking the original pain.

At the same time, the rubbing increases circulation in the underlying blood vessels, thereby warming the area and promoting healing.

Why do I feel better after taking a hot shower or bath?

Hot showers and baths are simple but effective therapeutic agents. For one thing, they relax the muscles, alleviating the pain associated with stress. For another, they increase the flow of blood to the extremities, easing discomfort in the joints. Lastly, they help stabilize one's heart rate and blood pressure.

Why do I have bad days and good days?

Whether you feel intense pain, relative pain, or no pain at all on a given day is based on the complex interaction of three factors. The first is your stamina, in terms of the physical and mental toughness you can bring to bear on your problem. A sleepless night practically guarantees a bad day. The second is pinpointing the actual cause of your discomfort and putting it in context. You can have "good" pain after surgery, as noted, because it indicates healing, but the "good" pain can cause a "bad" day. The third factor is understanding how your environment—the setting in which you live, work, play, and, yes, suffer—is helping or hindering your progress.

When you do have a bad day, you should carefully examine these factors—your stamina, the reason for your pain, your environment—with an eye toward taking a positive attitude about them. More often than not, it works.

One last word. Even healthy people have their ups and downs. So it's not surprising that pain sufferers have them, too. As long as your overall progress is upward, short-term lapses should be expected. Look on them as minor obstacles on the road to recovery.

Understanding Pain III

Why do I usually feel pain in only one area of my body at a time?

Your brain focuses on the pain with the greatest intensity. This does not necessarily mean that your brain is not sending out other pain signals, only that they are being blocked.

Are some parts of the body more sensitive to pain than others?

Some parts of the body have more nerve endings, or pain receptors, than others. Injury to any area containing an abundance of receptors produces a more intense pain. Such areas include the mouth, nasal passages, mucous membranes surrounding the eyes, and the genital and anal orifices.

Why does head pain seem worse than other types?

When you feel head pain, it is because of vascular congestion or muscle tension in the tissue around the brain, not in the brain itself.

Your head pain probably seems more severe because it is in the area of the body's command center. Subconsciously, you are giving your discomfort a higher priority than if it were, say, in an extremity.

What is the difference between a tension headache and a migraine?

Tension headaches, which are of muscular origin, are commonplace ailments. You get them when you're under stress or when you hold your head in an unnatural position for too long. You usually feel pressure beginning at the back of the head, then moving forward over the top of the head to the brow.

Migraines, which are of vascular origin, are rarer and more painful. They seem to be genetically inspired, often afflicting members of the same family. Instead of pressure, you feel a throbbing sensation.

Do damaged nerves ever heal?

Yes, but at a very slow rate and only after the agent causing the damage is removed. Severed nerves actually may have to be surgically repaired. The healing occurs on a microscopic level, and the return of normal function and sensation may take weeks, months, or even years.

We most often see damage to the outer layer of the nerve, which is called the myelin sheath. Undue pressure on the sheath results in such injuries as carpal tunnel syndrome.

As a rule of thumb, most doctors estimate that a severely damaged nerve at best takes an inch a month to recover. So a twelve-inch lesion requires a year of therapy, with the patient continually exercising the related muscle group until the nerve heals.

What fears do we harbor about pain?

One is that the discomfort will make life unbearable. But today we have such powerful and diverse painkillers that this concern is excessive and exaggerated.

Another is that the pain is signaling a life-threatening ailment or disease. Fortunately, in most cases, it is only alerting us to a problem.

We tell our patients: Don't let your pain control you. Put it in perspective.

Can excruciating pain cause death?

Intolerable pain, as noted, mercifully brings about a loss of consciousness. If such pain is not properly and promptly treated, however, it can cause various organ systems to malfunction, ultimately leading to death. The shock the pain inflicts on the body is just one element in a complex, and deadly, chain reaction.

If the brain is where pain is interpreted, why doesn't it feel pain?

The brain itself has no pain receptors. It is simply the storehouse of the pain experience, evaluating and transmitting all messages picked up by the nervous system.

Why do some minor injuries, like paper cuts, hurt so much?

Basically, most paper cuts are in the fingertip, where there is a greater number of nerve endings than in other areas. Because there are more of them, the brain gets a louder message.

Injuries in the extremities—hands and fingers, feet and toes—

also tend to be repetitive, since you're using them so often. You get one paper cut, then reopen it, aggravating the injury.

Does the anticipation of pain sometimes hurt as much as the actual pain?

Certainly. Your anticipation roils your emotions, reproducing pain based on previous experiences.

Does the body "remember" pain?

All unpleasant sensory stimuli flow into the brain's memory bank, often staying there after the cause of the discomfort has been removed. Proof of this is seen in phantom pain syndrome.

Do amputees experience pain?

Amputation may occur as a result of trauma or conditions such as diabetic disease. There may be pain at the actual site due to healing difficulties or vascular difficulties. However, another more elusive syndrome exists. "Phantom pain" may occur, which is pain sensed in parts of the limb that are no longer there. Phantom pain may sometimes be lessened by early prosthetic filling for the involved limb.

Why do some people who exercise believe "no pain, no gain"?

It's normal for us to experience small amounts of pain during and after exercise. Increased muscle use after relative inactivity, the buildup of lactic acid from the exertion, minor tearing in the muscle tissue—these factors cause mild discomfort. But, on the whole, our bodies benefit from working up a sweat.

The danger is in going overboard, accepting large amounts of pain. At a certain level, your pain receptors will tell you what you're doing is not right for someone of your age, physical condition, or skills. Listen to them.

When pain strikes, is it better to take a break or tough it out?

Once pain starts, there's no way of turning it back. You have to let it run its course, all the while alleviating it and, ultimately, preventing its recurrence.

That said, what usually determines whether you should rest is the pain's severity. The greater the discomfort, the more likely it is that you should take it easy.

With proper guidance from your doctor, you can develop an internal "thermostat," coming to understand which injuries and ailments require rest and which don't.

Understanding Pain IV

Why do some pains feel sharp and others dull, some stabbing and others throbbing?

The skin has various types of receptors. The kind of pain you feel depends on which nerve endings are triggered, and how forcefully. Sharp pains are associated with acute injury; dull ones, with chronic pain. Stabbing pains are linked to the nervous system; throbbing ones, to the vascular system.

Is it true there's a fine line between pleasure and pain?

Pleasure and *pain* are fundamental terms, and noted thinkers have discussed them in tandem through the ages, usually in terms of good versus evil. Medically speaking, the line between them is often one of degree. Initial pressure on swelling, for instance, will relieve the pain; continued pressure, cutting off the circulation, will worsen it.

It's true, too, that pleasure and pain can exist simultaneously. Numerous primitive rituals give testimony to this, right up to the present-day custom of body piercing.

We tend to agree with the philosopher John Locke, who said of the two emotions: "The way of knowing them . . . is only by experience."

Is there a link between pain and personality?

We strongly believe so. A negative attitude about life, fostering dark, brooding thoughts and the worst kind of introspection, only heightens one's discomfort. Studies have shown that the more optimistic people are, the stronger their immune system. Patients should continually remind themselves that the glass is half full, not half empty.

Does being in chronic pain raise your tolerance for future pain?

This is true in the sense that chronic pain can mask new and different types of pain. Your receptors, in effect, become overloaded by the continuous messages they are receiving.

Suppose the measurement of your chronic pain is at 7—on a scale of 0 to 10. If another painful stimulus strikes, chances are that you will not notice it unless the new sensation is greater than 7.

How does pain affect the immune system?

Let's take a moment to understand what the immune system is. When a disease-causing substance enters your body, it's confronted and normally put to rout by a host of immune cells—so-called B cells and T cells perhaps being the most prominent.

Sometimes, though, immune cells become hyperactive, mistaking healthy tissue for disease-causing invaders and bringing about such problems as arthritis, lupus, or diabetes. Or they become underactive—in the case of AIDS, for example.

Studies show that many of these longtime illnesses, with their attendant chronic pain, drastically alter and weaken the immune system. So it's reasonable to assume that pain plays a major role. Certainly such factors as emotional stress, poor diet, and lack of sleep—all of which intensify pain—reduce our resistance to disease.

Are failures in the immune system difficult to diagnose?

Decidedly so. The American Autoimmune Related Diseases Association reports that the average sufferer sees seven doctors over a five-year period before immune-system damage is identified. Resulting illnesses include rheumatoid arthritis, diabetes, multiple sclerosis, lupus, and psoriasis.

Why the body turns on itself, in effect mistaking its own cells for intruders, is unclear. Since autoimmunity is three times more common in women than in men, most theories focus on the unwise use of female hormones, especially estrogen.

We can do little at present to treat the various manifestations of immune-system failure. Nonsteroidal anti-inflammatories like ibuprofen or stronger prescription drugs may be given to patients, or immunosuppressants such as steroids may be recommended. The choice of drug and the extent of the dosage must be made on an individual basis.

Does chronic pain ever go away of its own accord?

In a sense. Because the severity of chronic pain can fluctuate and its duration is not predictable, the patient can be free (or relatively free) of pain for long periods.

Understand that there are two types of chronic pain. One is the acute-chronic, where the initial pain was caused by injury, but the discomfort persists, on and off, past the usual healing period. The other is the recurrent type, where pain begins gradually, with or without an identifiable cause, and subsides with or without treatment.

In both instances the danger is that patients will become fixated on their pain, prolonging their discomfort.

Pain is a symptom, but a most subjective one. It flows and ebbs, comes and goes, to a great extent in reaction to how you perceive it. That is why we treat a patient's psychological state as much as his or her physical one.

Does chronic pain ever go away for good?

It can. The epidemiology of pain, as noted, requires the interaction of three factors: (1) the state of your body, from both a psychological and physical standpoint; (2) the agent causing the pain, whether primary or secondary; and (3) the environment in which you live, ranging from climatic conditions to social relationships to economic security.

If we succeed in changing any one of these factors for the better, the chronic pain cycle can be broken.

As you get older, does chronic pain get better or worse?

There's no evidence that getting older necessarily worsens pain.

It's true that many older people do develop pain in their necks, shoulders, fingers, and lower backs from such ailments as osteoarthritis, nerve degeneration, osteoporosis, shortening of the tendons and muscles, and headaches. All these aches are examples of recurrent pain. But they are usually relatively mild and should be accepted as a normal part of the aging process. Going to extreme lengths to alleviate them is often not practical.

That said, it should be emphasized that chronic pain should not be allowed to plunge older people into depression. If it threatens to do so, doctors should make every effort to treat the pain as well as the depression.

Why do some injuries stay painful for so long?

You sprain your ankle and it supposedly heals. Then three months later the pain comes back. Probably it's a case of the tissues around the injury still being damaged and some exertion on your part irritating them again.

If you do not give the ankle the rest and treatment it needs, once and for all, the pain may well become an obsession, taking up an ever larger role in your life. By being impatient with the healing process, you are perpetuating the pain.

Can some forms of chronic pain be avoided by changing bad habits?

Definitely. Sometimes we prolong our pain simply by performing certain repetitive actions at work, at home, or in recreational settings in inefficient ways, not allowing the stressed parts of our anatomy to recover.

Work efficiency, for instance, calls for better positioning of computer keyboards, better sitting posture, better design of business forms. Home-environment efficiency involves raising and lowering cabinets and shelves, rearranging cooking areas, learning new house-cleaning techniques. Recreational efficiency requires using the proper type of athletic shoe, the right club or racquet, knowing the limits of one's stamina.

Can I learn more about pain management by surfing the Web?

You can certainly obtain access to a flood of information. Whether it applies specifically to your case or whether you are interpreting the medical reports and studies correctly may be open to debate. And yes, like most doctors, we readily admit to being put off by patients who confront us with a stack of printouts involving arcane or experimental research and expect us to make instant responses.

That said, we are also dedicated to the idea that patients who are well informed about their problems will be better able to cope with them. So we realize that the Web is here to stay. Perhaps the best of the on-line sources of medical information is Medline, which is part of the National Institutes of Health's National Library of Medicine. "Our major initiative now is trying to get information to the consumer," Eve-Marie Lacroix, chief of the public-services division of the library, recently stated.

Not only does Medline deal with individual ailments, but it provides medical encyclopedias and dictionaries to help viewers understand unfamiliar terms. Though the information is free of charge, much of it is available only in summary. To obtain the whole article, you may be required to pay a fee to various libraries and journals.

To help the patient better understand on-line medical data, the *New England Journal of Medicine* has joined with HealthGate Data Corporation (healthgate.com) to create *Weekly Briefings,* a summary of research from the *NEJM* written in laymen's language, including the reasons why a particular study was commissioned and how it was constructed.

"For most things there is no absolute answer," cautioned Jeffrey M. Drazen, editor in chief of the *NEJM* and professor of medicine at Harvard Medical School. "You might find a paper with an answer, but it might not be *the* answer."

Coping with Pain I

Is a sense of humor good medicine for pain?

Holding on to your sense of humor in adversity is always good medicine. Laughter helps relax the muscles, stimulate breathing, even produce more endorphins.

Can music soothe pain?

No doubt about it. Studies have shown, for instance, that patients listening to music they enjoy before, during, and after surgery demand fewer painkillers, thereby speeding the healing process.

What types of music therapy are there?

Music therapy includes simple listening, playing an instrument, composing music, even singing and chanting.

Listening's therapeutic qualities have to do with many musical elements. Tone, pitch, volume, and familiarity with the piece all determine how much the individual benefits. Strings may be preferred to woodwinds, brass to percussion.

Playing, with its manual skills, adds tactile qualities to the experience. Composing music, reverie. Singing and chanting, breath control and pacing.

Why do these therapies work? Understand that no greater or more complicated rhythms exist than those within our bodies. The musical rhythms somehow complement our biological ones, helping us transcend pain.

When I'm in love, my pain subsides. Why is this?

Your body undergoes positive changes in respiration, heart rate, and muscle relaxation. It probably even produces more endorphins.

We've discussed how negative feelings can increase your pain. Being in love is the other side of the emotional coin.

Why do I feel a compelling need to describe my pain to others?

Talking over a problem with professionals helps you understand it better. The whole process of psychotherapy consists of one person discussing his or her difficulty with another, objective individual. By sharing the experience, the patient also escapes the feeling of isolation that makes the discomfort so difficult to bear.

But a "compelling need" to talk to nonprofessionals may be a danger signal. You may be getting caught up in a self-pitying mode, trying to draw inordinate attention to your pain. This is understandable, but it is certainly counterproductive.

What qualities should I look for in a psychotherapist?

Just as important as your therapist's perceptiveness is the need that his or her responses be nonjudgmental. Otherwise, the two of you will not develop the required rapport to work out your problem.

What are "coping" strategies?

We learn practical ways to deal with pain, not only from doctors but from experience. We come to see that listening to music or meditation tapes relieves a headache. Or wearing well-designed shoes reduces foot pain. Or changing our behavior or taking warm baths eases a backache.

What does it mean to "ride the pain"?

It means facing up to your situation and continuing to live your life as normally as possible. By confronting your discomfort and refusing to let it embitter you, you at least eliminate its psychological damage. You go with the flow, you "ride the pain."

Suppose I feel pain coming on. What is the single most effective thing I can do to ease it?

Learn to relax. This advice is not as simple as it sounds, and you may need many sessions with a doctor or therapist, depending on your problem, before mastering the methods that work best for you.

Coping with Pain II

Why do I sometimes feel I'm in my own little world? How can I get out?

Feelings of isolation, with related depression, often develop in the crucible of chronic pain. Unless you fight your discomfort, it can envelop you, shutting you off from others, making you see yourself as worthless and unwanted.

To regain contact with the rest of the world, you must make the effort to communicate with it. Learn to put your suffering into words, to describe your pain in understandable terms, and—above all—not to perceive yourself as a victim.

Reaching out to family members and friends is the first step. If your feelings of isolation are severe, however, you need nonjudgmental, professional guidance.

On an immediate level, how can I deal with the anger and depression that result from chronic pain?

Recognize that it's not just the pain that's making you angry. It's the wondering when it will end, why the medication isn't working, whether you'll ever again get a good night's sleep—the "vicious cycle" discussed earlier.

You've got to break this cycle. How? Stop lamenting, "Why is this happening to *me?*" Start asking, "Why am *I* making this happen?" Understand that your problems must be attacked one by one. Your anger is normal. Your approach to dealing with it should be realistic.

How can I help a loved one in chronic pain?

Listen. Often sufferers do not need specific advice from relatives or friends as much as they need a sounding board. Sharing the experience of pain helps sufferers define their problems and begin working on positive solutions.

You should not expect to resolve your loved one's distress. Your encouragement will be therapy enough.

How can I keep pain from controlling my life?

By observing two virtues. First, live in the present, not the past or the future. Focus on the immediate causes of pain, those that can be controlled—not bitter memories or anticipated fears. Second, practice patience. Bear up, knowing that the trial will end. The result will be not growing dissatisfaction but growing peace of mind.

How can I turn my pain into something positive?

We train our patients to develop a methodology—a systematic body of procedures and techniques—to help them address their pain. Our aim is to remove the frustration from their lives. We do this by showing them how to score small but incremental successes.

Take the length of the day. People suffering pain at sporadic intervals can easily come to feel that they're constantly in pain. But they're not. So we tell them to divide the day into segments—hours and half hours. Then they can see for themselves their good and bad times.

Simultaneously, and depending on the patient's ailment, we suggest appropriate coping and relaxation techniques. Every program is individually designed. With each small step forward, patients feel more positive about themselves.

Once people achieve these initial successes, they are positioning themselves for larger ones.

What are some of the major advances in the treatment and diagnosis of pain?

Certain alternative treatments are coming into their own. Acupuncture, for instance, is winning more and more converts, at least for short-term relief. In this procedure, which may help produce more endorphins, trained therapists insert hair-thin needles through the skin, trying to channel the body's neural impulses into the healing process.

Similarly, acupressure is increasingly popular. This technique, which can be self-applied, calls for brief, steady pressure at the site of an ailment and, often, at several bodily points leading to and away from it.

Thermal biofeedback is a third intriguing alternative treatment. Effective in reducing stress, it involves the use of escalating amounts of heat to the hands and feet.

Meanwhile, a host of technological advances have made pinpointing pain, and therefore diagnosing it, more and more accurate. Position emission tomography (PET) scans use radioactive imaging to detect problems in the brain and heart. Magnetic resonance imaging (MRI) procedures employ magnetic imaging to find defects throughout the body, while CAT (computed tomography) scans use computer-enhanced X rays for the same purpose.

I've heard that PET scans and MRI procedures can now actually let the doctor look into the brain and "see" pain at work as it "lights up" specific neutrons. Is this true?

Great strides have been made, but far more work has to be done. Scientists at the State University of New York's Health Science Center in Syracuse, for instance, have used functional MRIs (fMRIs) to locate cell groups in the cerebral cortex that are activated by severe pain in the hands, back muscles, and spinal cord tissues. Such research, while still in the preliminary stage, debunks the old notion that it is less important to treat the pain than the underlying disease. The fact is that pain, like blood pressure, can now be measured.

The SUNY researchers used fMRI machines to send radio waves into the brain, where they interacted with hydrogen atoms to "light up" the neutrons responding to the pain. All the patients with hand problems showed similar patterns in the brain, and those with back-muscle and spinal-cord problems showed varying patterns. Not only was the degree of pain measured, but its location in the cerebral cortex was pinpointed.

How can I best take advantage of these and other advances?

It's essential to know the exact level of training, licensing, and experience of the doctor who's treating your pain. Similarly, you should know the exact level of technology that's available at the clinic where he or she is practicing.

You can obtain information about pain-control centers through directories and databases maintained at hospitals, support groups for various illnesses (e.g., the Arthritis Foundation or the Multiple Sclerosis Society), or even community centers.

Other referrals may come from your family doctor, personal recommendations, or the Internet. Check them out carefully, then take advantage of them.

Do we still need to know more about pain?

Our biggest problem with pain is that its essential causation—from patient to patient—remains amorphous. Some people report severe discomfort, and the doctor knows they are hurting but cannot readily find a cause. Other people who have major physical problems, such as slipped discs, show little discomfort. This is why we say all pain is individual.

In some instances, pain is a psychological experience; in others, a physical one. The boundaries between these worlds are indistinct. Meanwhile, the art of pain management lies in helping the patient interpret the two overlapping spheres.

Will my health insurance cover pain management?

You'll have to read your policy carefully, relate its coverage to your symptoms, and then, to make sure of the coverage, contact your insurance representative.

Be prepared to answer specific questions: Is this a new diagnosis? Have you been previously covered for a related ailment? Will the examination or treatment be done on an outpatient or inpatient basis?

If you have a grasp of these issues, you'll be better prepared to negotiate your coverage with your insurance provider.

Are there advocates who can help me deal with my insurer?

One source of help is typified by the Patient Advocate Foundation, a nonprofit organization based in Newport News, Virginia. Not only does it have a nationwide network, but it doesn't hesitate to apply pressure to insurers if it feels they are dragging their feet on needed procedures, including those for pain management. The PAF can be reached through its Web site at www.patient advocate.org, or by phone at 800-532-5274. Nancy Davenport-Ennis, its founder and executive director, recently declared, "We became the coach on how to get through the appeals process for the sick patient who says, 'I'm exhausted, I can't take the battle with my insurance company or my employer.' "

Hospitals often provide a second type of support, assigning staff members to help people wade through the paperwork demanded by insurers and employers in such areas as insurance claims, managed care, and treatment delays.

How prevalent are disputes over coverage for pain management?

Unfortunately, such disputes parallel those for medical coverage in general. One study by the Kaiser Family Foundation and the Harvard School of Public Health recently found that 87 percent of doctors surveyed reported some kind of denial of coverage by health plans.

Another study, by Kaiser and *Consumer Reports*, concluded that 50 percent of patients surveyed had had a significant problem with their health insurance.

How can I best deal with my insurance company regarding the cost of pain management?

Once again, proper preparation is the key. Often certain procedures must be approved in advance to get proper reimbursement. Other times inpatient admissions may require that various criteria be met. If you make an effective case, usually you can reach an accommodation with your insurer.

In the unhappy event that your policy does not cover treatment, the wiser course may be for you—in the earlier, more reversible stages of an ailment—to absorb the cost. This makes more sense than letting the ailment worsen and risking lengthy unemployment.

Conquering Pain I

None of the doctors I've seen have helped me. What else can I try?

So-called alternative therapies are coming more and more into the medical mainstream. Or they are being used in combination with traditional treatment. We have already mentioned music therapy, acupuncture, acupressure, and thermal biofeedback. Other alternative options include herbal medicine, aromatherapy, massage, yoga, guided imagery, hypnosis, and TENS (transcutaneous electrical nerve stimulation).

How prominent a group, within the medical profession, are the doctors who specialize in treating pain?

Over the past two decades, first dozens, now thousands of doctors have devoted their practices to managing pain. Currently physicians with specific training in this area are becoming board-certified. Various societies and publications, including the *International Journal of Pain Therapy*, have sprung up, and both large and small pain clinics have become commonplace in cities.

Our own affiliation, the Rusk Institute for Rehabilitation Medicine in New York City, is the oldest and largest such pain-management center, offering, we feel, the widest and most advanced array of services.

Still, we are a relatively young specialty. We do not even have sole claim to a medical name—as do obstetricians, urologists, and cardiologists. Our name, algologist, coming from *algos,* the Greek word for "pain," also describes scientists studying algae, from the Latin word for "seaweed." A humbling thought.

What tools are used to diagnose pain?

When patients first come to us, we ask them to fill out questionnaires on which they identify, insofar as they are able, the cause of their pain, its severity, and its duration. Then, as part of the therapeutic process, we have them keep detailed self-measurements, on a scale of 0 to 10, so that we can determine where, when, and for how long the discomfort occurs.

On the technological front, we use X rays, MRIs, and CAT scans to find and treat probable trouble spots. Some devices, such as thermographs, even help us measure an individual's sensitivity.

What you should bear in mind, however, is that all these tools, or at least their interpretation, are essentially subjective. Long-term relief of chronic pain, in the final analysis, depends on the skill and experience of the diagnostician.

How is pain affected by diet?

You will be far better able to cope with pain if your body is in the best shape possible—considering your age and ailments. This means you shouldn't (1) carry around excess weight, (2) clog your arteries with needless fats, (3) avoid high-fiber fruits and vegetables, (4) scarf down sweets, (5) use too much salt, or (6) drink too much alcohol. Moderation, we repeat, in all things.

How is pain affected by exercise?

Exercise would ease pain if for no other reason than it gets the sufferers out of themselves and into the physical world. But exercise's efficacy goes beyond that. For one thing, the exertion produces more endorphins, whose opiate-like effect reduces pain. For another, working up a sweat increases the circulation rate, leading to relaxation and warmth.

Anybody can exercise. You needn't be Mr. or Ms. Total Fitness, or even go to a health club. For instance, lie down on your back on the floor, stretch your arms over your head, and instantly feel the tension leaving your body. Then stretch the muscles in your stomach, your buttocks, your calves and experience the same feeling in those areas. Then exhale deeply, suck in your stomach, press the small of your back against the floor, and notice how good your back feels.

How is pain affected by sleeplessness?
Sleep deprivation leads to anxiety, irritability, and depression, psychological states that greatly weaken the body's resistance to pain.

Don't rely on medications to get a good night's sleep. Instead, rely on regular habits.

Suggestions: Don't drink alcohol or caffeine for several hours before bedtime. Exercise, by all means, but during the day, not before retiring. Take a hot shower or bath before turning in. Read or meditate for a few minutes, or have a warm drink, before calling it a day. Don't go to bed if you aren't sleepy, but do get up at the same time each morning, even if you've had a bad night.

How is pain affected by alcohol or caffeine?
The use of alcohol or caffeine temporarily lessens pain, but hours later, once the effect of either substance wears off, chances are that you'll feel much worse.

Alcohol, a relaxant, causes vascular dilation, temporarily creating a sense of well-being and relieving such ailments as hypertension. Caffeine, a stimulant, brings about vascular contraction, in the short run easing the pain, say, of a migraine.

Overreliance on either substance leads, at best, to irritability; at worse, to belligerent or even violent behavior.

How can I live with stress and still control my pain?

In the long term, working with your doctor or therapist, you should utilize such techniques as relaxation exercises, hypnotherapy, and guided imagery. In the short term, act positively. Divide your days into quadrants or hours, enjoying your "good" times and resolving to reduce your "bad" times.

Does the weather affect pain?

Very much so. A sure sign that bad weather is coming and that the barometer is falling is increased pain in arthritic joints. A surge in humidity often brings headaches, as well as sinus and neck discomfort. Lengthy rainfall contributes to depression, as do shorter hours of daylight; both abet suicidal impulses. Allergens and pollution particles in the air clearly cause respiratory problems.

When is surgery necessary to stop pain?

Sometimes the simple removal, for example, of the appendix, gallbladder, or tumors will stop pain by relieving obstruction, compression, or infection. But other sources of pain, and their causes, are more difficult to find.

Take care not to rush into surgery until you feel that your doctor has identified the precise cause of your pain. If you're in any doubt, get a second opinion. This will ensure not only that the operation is a success but that your postsurgical recovery is total.

What is "guided imagery"?

This is a technique often used to reduce and control pain. We show patients a positive image, perhaps a flower in full bloom or a glorious sunrise. We then "guide" them into concentrating on the image so that the picture helps them forget—temporarily, at least—the source of their discomfort.

Focusing on the flower or the sunrise, patients immerse themselves in the beauty, warmth, and color of the image, pushing their pain into the background. Hope replaces gloom.

Can hypnosis relieve pain?

Definitely, although the success rate may vary, depending on the skill of the therapist and the cooperation of the patient.

Hypnosis is a good management option for people who suffer from chemical intolerance, or for people who are chemically addicted, thereby limiting their medication options.

The Spiegel (eye-roll) Test measures susceptibility to hypnotic suggestion.

Conquering Pain II

Do all people experience pain?

A group of people have been identified who experience a congenital absence of pain. The state is associated with a lifelong tendency to cuts, burns, and injury because the individual is unable to experience pain and learn to protect the body from trauma.

What are the principal medications used to relieve pain?

There are two categories. One is opioid analgesics, commonly called narcotics. All are in one way or another related to morphine, which is derived from opium poppies. Narcotics attack the brain and the neural system and are quite effective in treating severe pain, but they pose significant addictive risks.

The second, less powerful category is nonopioid analgesics, the first of which was aspirin, originally derived from tree bark. Nonopioid analgesics attack the site of the pain. Almost all are anti-inflammatory, allowing the injury to heal while reducing its pain. Anti-inflammatory drugs other than aspirin are less likely to produce such aspirin-like side effects as stomach irritation.

Within these two categories, there are literally hundreds of choices.

How does my doctor decide which medication is best for me?

Doctors make this decision based on several factors, the most important being the patient's age and medical history, the severity of pain, and the degree of risk.

Often what is right for one patient is not right for another. Even when a medication is helpful, its effectiveness should be continually monitored.

Isn't this whole business about continually monitoring medications a stratagem on the part of my doctor to keep me coming back?

Not at all. Modern-day medications are a blessing to us all, often curing or at least arresting disease and eliminating the need for surgery. But the other side of the coin is that these drugs are incredibly complicated, chemically speaking, and work in the body in complicated ways. Consider Vioxx, a nonsteroidal anti-inflammatory drug (NSAID) that is used to ease swelling and soreness. In its advertisements the company making the drug points out that Vioxx relieves (1) osteoarthritis, the disease caused by wear and tear on bones and joints; (2) the short-term pain following dental or surgical operations; and (3) menstrual pain.

But in the very same ads, the pharmaceutical company rightly lays out a wide spectrum of cautions. Do not take Vioxx, it stresses, if you have had allergic reactions such as asthma or hives. Tell your doctor, the company goes on to say, if you are planning to become pregnant or are breast-feeding, because Vioxx may harm the fetus or infant. Additionally, it warns, before taking the medication, tell your doctor if you have kidney or liver disease, high blood pressure, or serious stomach problems or if you experience a sharp weight gain or swelling in your arms or legs.

Vioxx is for most users presumably a safe drug, one approved by the Food and Drug Administration. But the cautions about its proper use, issued by the company making it, go on and on. So you can see that most patients, particularly those who are in discomfort, are in no position to make detached decisions about whether to begin taking such a drug and when to stop taking it.

The long and the short of it is that patients taking strong medication need careful monitoring. Informed physicians are knowledgeable about the plethora of drugs available, match them to sufferers' ever changing needs, and keep the wellness train on track. Treat yourself and you may find yourself going off the rails.

Are some painkillers harmful?

Great care must be taken in prescribing all painkillers. Narcotic drugs, for instance, present clear addictive problems, although these concerns, in the case of the terminally ill, may well give way to the greater good of easing the patient's pain.

Dependence, even on over-the-counter drugs, should be shunned. Painkillers are meant to help you through a difficult, but finite, period, not become a way of life.

When taking such medication, patients should tell their doctors about any adverse physical reactions, behavioral changes, or mood swings they may encounter.

Can you name some specific painkillers?

Understand that the following examples are generalizations. Even the over-the-counter medications should be taken with care; prescription drugs should be constantly supervised.

For *mild* discomfort: Tylenol, an acetaminophen, is usually well tolerated but should not be taken over the long term by patients with liver and kidney problems. Aspirin, an acetylsalicylic acid, is comparable to Tylenol but is more likely to produce a burning sensation, particularly in those who have ulcers or other stomach conditions. Nor should aspirin be given to children for flu symptoms or chicken pox.

Nonsteroidal anti-inflammatory drugs such as Motrin, Advil, and Aleve are also effective in treating mild pain. They basically are for young, healthy adults whose symptoms require only occasional relief. They should not be taken casually by the elderly or by high-risk individuals with chronic problems.

For *moderate* discomfort: Vicodin or Lortab, which are hydrocodones-acetaminophens, may be the best in their class and are more powerful and less constipating than codeine. Hydrocodones are particularly effective in easing muscle and bone pain. Tylenol #3, acetaminophen with codeine, in our view runs second in this category.

For *severe* discomfort: Dilaudid, a short-acting narcotic pain reliever, produces a euphoric effect and is used in treating cancer patients. Morphine sulphate, an even stronger drug, is administered to individuals whose pain is incapacitating.

How do painkillers become addictive?

Usually through overuse. The body develops an ever greater tolerance for the drug, demanding ever greater amounts. We call this a chemical addiction, and attempts at withdrawal bring about obvious physical changes in one's vital signs (such as heart rate and blood pressure) and mood.

Behavioral addiction is less common. The user becomes emotionally dependent upon the medication but does not display the classic signs of withdrawal.

If painkillers are not harmful or addictive, can they ever be inappropriate therapy?

Yes, if they mask a pain symptom instead of allowing one to heed it. People suffering from acute appendicitis, for example, require immediate medical attention. Giving them painkillers instead of performing surgery would be wrong. You would, in effect, be turning off the body's alarm system.

Painkillers are also inappropriate if they bring about allergic reactions or associated side effects like gastrointestinal upset, respiratory distress, and rash.

How exactly do our bodies produce endorphins, or natural painkillers?

Endorphins are hormones that combine with opiates in the brain, usually in times of great stress, to relieve pain. These hormones come from the anterior lobe of the tiny pituitary gland, the so-called master gland located at the base of the brain. Once in the bloodstream, the pituitary's secretions directly affect our sensitivity to pain.

What is the role of adrenaline in reducing pain?

Adrenaline does not so much relieve or neutralize pain as alert our bodies to danger, giving us the choice of "flight or fight." Surges of adrenaline, which is also a hormone, frequently occur when one is threatened or challenged. In this case, the secretions come from the adrenal glands, located above the kidneys. These surges quickly intensify heartbeat, breathing, and blood flow into the muscles, often enabling ordinary people to perform extraordinary physical feats.

Conquering Pain III

How does acupuncture work?

Hairlike needles are gently inserted into the skin along pathways traditionally thought to channel energy through the body. Where precisely they are placed depends on where the pain is.

This technique (1) speeds up the production of endorphins; (2) releases serotonins and other chemicals into the bloodstream, increasing circulation; (3) at least temporarily relieves muscle spasms; and (4) produces steroidlike substances that reduce inflammation.

Is acupuncture safe?

Properly performed, the procedure is quite safe, but like all treatments, damage can result if it is administered by inexperienced practitioners. There are some nine thousand licensed acupuncturists in the United States, performing millions of procedures annually. Thirty-six states and the District of Columbia require licensing, while eleven other states have such legislation pending. Additionally, some seven thousand physicians in the United States have taken postgraduate training in acupuncture.

The most common major injury is a collapsed lung, caused when a needle penetrates too deeply; the most common minor injuries are bruising, bleeding, and soreness. The onetime bane of acupuncture, a hepatitis B or C infection, has all but disappeared because of the use of sterile, disposable needles. No hepatitis cases have been reported since 1988.

What conditions are usually treated by acupuncture?

Two of the most prevalent are low back pain and headache. It is also used in the treatment of pain associated with surgery and nausea following chemotherapy.

How does acupressure work?

Therapists (and, for that matter, patients) use hand pressure, instead of needles, along the same acupuncture pathways.

The disadvantage of this procedure is that its effect is less powerful than acupuncture. The advantages are that patients, properly trained, can treat themselves and that, for the squeamish, it is needle-free.

How effective is TENS (transcutaneous electrical nerve stimulation)?

This therapy, which involves passing a mild electrical current through the skin by means of a small transmitter, thereby stimulating the nerves, can be quite beneficial. Used by prescription and under the direction of a clinician, it enables patients to ease their pain in their own homes, at any hour of the day or night.

It should be acknowledged, however, that TENS is more effective in relieving minor discomfort than major problems.

What is biofeedback?

It's a system of pain control designed to give patients information about how their bodies are reacting to pain. Using computers, we monitor such vital functions as heart rate, brain waves, blood pressure, and skin temperature to create a total physiological picture.

We give patients "feedback," through printouts and displays, so they understand how their bouts with pain are affecting their bodies. Our hope is that they will then be better able to modify and control their reactions.

Can breathing exercises relieve pain?

Pain reduction can be achieved simply by changing your breathing pattern. When a pain attack strikes, resist the compulsion to breathe rapidly and shallowly. Concentrate on breathing slowly and deeply.

Can massage?

Yes. Massage increases blood circulation in the muscles, carrying away harmful products that tend to irritate the nerve endings and generally relaxing the body. Simultaneously, the laying-on of hands has an overall healing effect.

Still, we should recognize that massage is a passive procedure, not a substitute for the total benefits achieved through exercise.

Can yoga?

Yoga can definitely play a role in pain reduction. The ritual, involving slow and sustained body positions and movements, promotes muscle stretching, spinal and limb flexing, and general relaxation. But to be fully effective, yoga requires considerable guidance and training.

Can vitamin supplements alleviate pain?

Only in the sense that any nutritional imbalance weakens the body, making it more susceptible to pain-related illness. If you are not getting enough folic acid, for instance, you could be developing neurological impairment and heightening your sensitivity to pain. But before rushing out and buying some vitamin B complex/folic acid capsules, consider eating more green, leafy salads and fresh fruit—foods rich in folic acid.

What is herbal medicine?

This therapy involves a potpourri of preparations, made from herbs and plants, that are thought to cure or at least alleviate various ailments. Herbal doses can be taken internally—in teas, water extracts, and tinctures—or applied externally, in poultices, ointments, or powders.

Precisely because herbs do have medicinal properties, great care should be exercised in how they are used.

Can herbal medicines do as much harm as good?

Herbal medicines, like all medications, can be misapplied and abused. That is why patients should not diagnose themselves.

- St.-John's-wort, for instance, may be of benefit for depression but may be counterproductive and even dangerous for those with HIV infections and organ transplants.

- Saw palmetto seems to relieve prostate enlargement, but long-term studies are needed before this can be shown with certainty.

- Ginseng likewise appears to have antioxidant qualities that inhibit types of cell damage associated with artery disease and aging, but we do not know whether the herb is safe for cancer patients.

- Comfrey, thought to be useful in treating inflammation and constipation, may contribute to liver failure.

- Garlic, eaten cooked or raw, may decrease the risk of stomach cancer, but garlic supplements are next to useless.

- Ginkgo biloba may slow mental decline, but in no way does it improve memory.

To sum up: Some herbs may be beneficial to some people, but professional advice should be sought before taking them.

What are homeopathic drugs?

Homeopathic remedies, while also prepared from herbs and plants, are not to be confused with herbal medicine.

Most homeopathic dosages are prepared, in extremely diluted form, from poisonous substances. The theory, which is two hundred years old, is that if a substance, in its pure form, can produce unhealthy symptoms in a healthy person, then the same substance, diluted, can reverse those symptoms in an unhealthy person.

How risky are homeopathic drugs, and alternative therapies in general?

Homeopathic solutions are traditionally low-risk, but not risk-free. Preexisting medical factors, such as diabetes, hypertension, and immune dysfunction, may make a person extremely vulnerable to such drugs.

All alternative solutions, like those of traditional medicine, are only as effective as the skill and knowledge of the practitioner.

Part Three

Specific Problems

Abdominal Pain—Stomach (heartburn, gastroenteritis, irritable bowel syndrome, hernia, peptic ulcers)

How does heartburn differ from gastroenteritis?

Heartburn is caused by excessive acid in the abdominal area, usually as a result of overeating or eating too fast, and produces pain in the stomach and a burning sensation in the chest. Most heartburn cases can be relieved with over-the-counter antacids, but they should be used sparingly since they address only the symptoms, not the causes.

Gastroenteritis, sometimes called stomach flu, is caused by an infection in the digestive system, either bacterial or viral, and results in severe diarrhea. Over-the-counter drugs containing bismuth subsalicylate can be beneficial, but if the condition does not improve, your doctor will prescribe more powerful medications.

What are the best ways to avoid these problems?

To avoid heartburn: (1) eat wisely, reducing your intake of fatty foods, citrus fruits, garlic, onions, coffee, and alcohol; (2) eat slowly; and (3) avoid smoking.

To avoid bacterial gastroenteritis: (1) wash your hands often throughout the day; (2) take proper precautions in preparing and storing food at home; and (3) eat only in restaurants and fast-food outlets with proper sanitary standards. In the case of viral gastroenteritis, understand that the disease, which spreads quickly through large groups in close quarters, can be unavoidable; luckily, the symptoms usually abate within forty-eight hours.

What is irritable bowel syndrome (IBS), and what causes it?

It's a condition in which one's bowel movements for weeks on end are abnormal, usually resulting in stomach cramps, bloating, and diarrhea after meals, or, more rarely, constipation.

We don't really know what causes IBS, but we theorize that the condition may be triggered by a dietary imbalance, an intolerance for certain foods, or stress.

How is IBS treated?

First, we make sure the patient's diet contains enough fiber, ranging from whole grains to fresh fruit to green, leafy vegetables. We also restrict the intake of foods that irritate the digestive tract—fats, oils, spices, dairy products, and coffee. If the patient smokes, we urge him or her to quit. Simultaneously, we look for food intolerances.

Lastly, to calm the patient's digestion, we prescribe plenty of exercise—walking briskly, jogging, or swimming.

What about alternative therapies?

Biofeedback techniques can be effective in reducing tension, as can guided imagery and hypnotherapy.

How do abdominal hernias occur?

A weak spot in the muscle wall gives way, allowing an internal organ or tissue to push through the hole. The vast majority of abdominal hernias are inguinal, occurring among men, with part of the small intestine protruding into the groin, producing an obvious lump.

Such hernias can be quite painful, particularly when lifting, stretching, or coughing.

What remedies exist?

Surgery is the optimal treatment. The invasive tissue is pushed back, the muscle wall gets repaired, and the patient is discharged the next day. Work generally can be resumed within a week, and the incision is completely healed in a matter of months.

What's the latest surgical technique for repairing hernias?

Using mesh to repair the hole in the muscle wall seems to be more effective than simply using stitches. Surgeons implant a mesh patch in the hole, permitting new flesh growth and scar tissue to fill the gap. According to a recent study published in the *New England Journal of Medicine,* patients treated with mesh were only half as likely to suffer hernia recurrences within three years after surgery.

What are peptic ulcers?

They are literally holes, caused by excessive digestive acids, in the lining of the stomach. The most common are duodenal, found at the beginning of the small intestine just below the stomach, and gastric, in the stomach itself.

Sufferers experience burning pain, particularly after drinking coffee or alcohol.

What causes ulcers?

We used to think that the acid buildup was due exclusively to stress and an overreliance on stimulants. Now we see that bacterial infections may play a role, as well as the use of analgesics over a lengthy period.

Are there effective therapies?

In most cases, drugs called histamine blockers heal the holes in the stomach's lining within weeks. To combat infection, antibiotics may be prescribed.

Can you recommend some of these drugs?

If your ulcer is caused by an infection, it is treated with antibiotics and so-called pump blockers. Your doctor may prescribe a combination of Biaxin (which is clarithromycin), Prilosec (which is omeprazole), and Flagyl (which is metronidazole) over a ten-day period.

If your ulcer results not from infection but from irritation in the stomach lining, your physician may recommend Prilosec alone. This drug almost completely blocks acid production in the stomach. Prevacid is another possible remedy. In almost all cases such ulcers are eliminated within a four-week period.

What about diet?

Be abstemious in your intake of coffee, alcohol, and tobacco and extremely moderate in your consumption of everything else. Here's a tip: avoid milk. You may think it's "coating" your ulcer, but it's actually creating more acid.

Abdominal Pain—Other (kidney stones, gallstones, colitis, Crohn's disease, diverticulitis, endometriosis)

How do kidney stones differ from gallstones?

Kidney stones occur when chemicals in the urine crystallize in the ureter, blocking the flow of liquid from the bladder. Severe pain is felt in the side and groin.

Gallstones occur when chemicals crystallize in the gallbladder, the organ that stores bile—the liver's digestive juice. As long as the stone stays in the bladder, there is no problem. But if the stone leaves the bladder and gets stuck in the bile duct, severe pain is experienced in the right abdomen.

Kidney stones form mainly in the young and the early middle-aged, while gallstones, which for the most part affect women, form mainly in the late middle-aged.

What diagnostic tests are employed?

Common tests to locate kidney stones include special X rays and ultrasonic scanning. Tests to find gallstones include ultrasonic scanning, CTs (computerized tomography), and MRIs (magnetic resonance imaging).

How are these problems treated?

Most kidney stones exit the ureter on their own within days or weeks, so the usual therapy calls for drinking lots of water—several quarts a day—and taking painkillers. Heat can also be beneficial.

In more complicated cases, a sound-wave machine called a lithotripter is used to break up the stone, making it easier for the fragments to exit, or it is surgically removed.

Gallstone therapy is similar, calling for painkillers and a wait-

and-see approach, on the chance that the obstruction will leave the bile duct on its own. Bile salts may also be prescribed, to dissolve the stone.

Should these approaches fail, the lithotripter may be used; or the entire gallbladder, since it's not essential for a normal life, is excised.

If people are prone to these illnesses, what preventive measures can they take?

For kidney stones, drink plenty of water and, under professional supervision, learn how to avoid foods high in uric acid and calcium oxalate, which are stone-forming substances.

Gallstone attacks often can be forestalled by following a low-fat, high-fiber diet.

Can exercise help?

It certainly seems to in the case of gallstone attacks, two-thirds of which affect women. A recent Harvard School of Public Health study reported that women who exercise as little as thirty minutes a day cut their risk of gallstones by nearly one-third compared with women who do not work out.

The Harvard researchers speculate that exercise may reduce the cholesterol content of bile. This in turn reduces the number of gallstones, which are mostly solid cholesterol. Additionally, people who work out usually have more active large intestines and better levels of blood sugar and insulin, further lessening the risk of gallstone attacks.

The study also found that women who sit for forty to sixty hours a week are 42 percent more likely to need their gallbladders removed than those who spend most of their waking hours moving about. Women who sit for more than sixty hours a week are an astronomical 132 times more likely to require surgery.

What is colitis, and how serious is it?

This condition is a chronic inflammation of the large intestine, resulting in bloody diarrhea and abdominal pain. (It is sometimes confused with Crohn's disease, a similar inflammation with like symptoms, but one that affects the entire digestive tract.)

Ulcerative colitis is quite serious and, left untreated, can lead to colon cancer.

How is the condition handled?

Hydrocortisones are prescribed to alleviate the inflammation, along with drugs like loperamide to stop the diarrhea. Once the symptoms are arrested, the patient is put on a high-fiber diet and urged to exercise. (Crohn's disease, in contrast, cannot be cured, only controlled through drugs and, in extreme cases, surgery.)

You say Crohn's disease cannot be cured. Are there any experimental therapies on the horizon?

Human growth hormone combined with a high-protein diet significantly reduced the pain of three-quarters of patients on a short-term basis, according to a study published in the *New England Journal of Medicine*. The lead researcher of the piece, Dr. Alfred Slonim of North Shore University Hospital in Manhasset, New York, stressed that further research would be needed before growth hormone could be proved effective in the long term. If so, Dr. Slonim said, it may be safer than other therapies.

Some one million Americans suffer from Crohn's disease, which is diagnosed in as many as 120,000 people yearly.

Is diverticulitis still another inflammation of the intestines?

Yes, but one in which food or fecal matter gets caught in a series of bulges, or weak spots, in the intestine linings which then becomes infected. Pain on the left side of the abdomen and diarrhea result.

Who are most at risk?

Middle-aged people who eat a high-fat, low-fiber diet are the most likely victims. Experts estimate that half of all Americans, at some point in their lives, will suffer a diverticular attack. That's not an encouraging dietary statistic.

What are the usual therapies?

Antibiotics to control the infection, then the oft-mentioned need to ingest high-fiber foods. In chronic cases, surgery may be necessary.

What is endometriosis, and what part does it play in female infertility?

This problem occurs when bits of endometrial tissue, normally found only in the uterus, somehow find their way back through the fallopian tubes into the abdomen. There they stick to the ovaries and uterine ligaments, bleeding during menstruation just as if they were still in the uterus.

What results, besides abdominal pain, irritation, and scarring, is interference with the ovulation process. Studies indicate endometriosis is responsible for one-third of all female failure to conceive.

How is the disease treated?

Estrogens and progestins, among other drugs, are used to slow the growth of endometrial tissue. If surgery is needed, existing tissue can be removed during a laparoscopy, in which the doctor, through a small incision, inspects the abdominal cavity.

Which women are most likely to have this problem?

Women may be most susceptible if endometriosis runs in the family, menstrual periods are overlong, discharges are overly heavy, or tampons are not frequently changed.

I have heard that microcameras are being developed that patients will swallow to help doctors explore the abdominal cavity and digestive tract. Is this a spoof?

An Israeli company is seeking to market a pill-size radio camera, an inch long and half an inch wide, that after ingestion makes its way through the digestive tract, transmitting pictures all the time. The microdevice, which consists of a camera, light source, radio transmitters, and batteries, is being promoted as a minimally invasive way of viewing the small intestine. The batteries last some six hours, enough time for natural stomach contractions to move the device through the stomach. Patients do not have to interrupt their normal routines during the twenty-four to forty-eight hours the pills are in their digestive tracts before being excreted.

The camera transmits several images a second to a receiver the size of a Walkman that is attached around the patient's waist. The images are stored in memory chips and later downloaded to a computer for viewing. The manufacturer claims that these images will enable surgeons, for instance, to pinpoint the exact spot in the small intestine where they would have to operate.

Preliminary reports on the device recently appeared in the journal *Nature*. The manufacturer is Given Imaging of Yokneam, Israel, which is asking marketing approval from the U.S. Food and Drug Administration. "Once it's gone down, you don't feel it at all," stated Dr. Paul Swain, a gastroenterologist at the Royal London Hospital who conducted the initial trials.

After viewing a demonstration, Dr. James T. Frakes, past president of the American Society of Gastroenterologists, called the microcamera "a landmark event," adding that "the possibilities are limitless."

Abscesses

What are abscesses?

They are encapsulated pockets of pus, or dead white blood cells, caused by bacterial infections.

What are the symptoms?

Symptoms include pain, swelling, and fever. Abscesses in or below the skin produce visible swelling and redness. They whiten just before they burst, because they are stretching the skin.

Abscesses deep in the body often grow quite large before symptoms appear, and they can spread considerable infection. Luckily, X rays and MRIs (magnetic resonance imaging) do a good job of finding them.

Where are they likely to develop?

Just about anywhere; at skin level, especially in the face.

How are abscesses treated?

Lancing them lets out the accumulated pus and helps drain further secretions. The healing process is accelerated by antibiotics and frequently changed dressings.

Accidental Injuries

When do most accidental injuries occur?

Usually when you are participating in exertions that are either new or infrequently performed. Hence the relatively high incidence of injuries during vacations or recreational activities.

You may be at risk even at work, however, if you try to do too many things too fast under the stress of a deadline.

What precautions can I take while I'm on vacation?

It's not unusual for people on vacation to try new sports with either no training or minimal instruction—parasailing or scuba diving, snowboarding or ice skating. This is a recipe for disaster.

Similarly, keep in mind that you need the proper clothing and equipment, even for so simple an activity as prolonged walking or hiking.

Try to plan ahead, avoiding the unexpected.

What is the weekend warrior syndrome?

Career-oriented people are equally driven in their sports activities. They think they can go, effortlessly, from a sedentary job during the week to a strenuous sport on the weekend. They cannot. Because their muscles, coordination, and timing are not prepped for optimal performance, their chance of injury is high.

Recently we read a story about a young working mother who decided to join a kickboxing class. At 9 A.M. one Sunday morning, in a group of two dozen women, she suddenly found herself in constant and violent motion. "One, two, three, kick, punch, kick, kick, kick" was the way she described the scene, emphasizing the frenzied repetition of the drills. "The more you sweat, the better the workout," she enthused.

The young woman managed to get through the class in one piece, and she certainly enjoyed it, but her choice was a risky one. Weekend warriors, if they want to stay out of doctors' waiting rooms, should be more moderate in their activities. The idea is to follow a well-designed exercise program all through the week, one that safely conditions and stretches the muscles and pumps the vascular system.

Courting excitement is courting danger.

What other factors increase the risk of injury?

Although we innately seek someone or something to blame, injuries are a part of being mobile. Still, some decisions invite trouble:

- playing, working, or living in areas made hazardous by poor lighting, slippery surfaces, or atmospheric pollutants

- using the wrong or defective equipment, whether it be sports gear, tools, or home appliances

- overestimating one's athletic abilities and preparedness

- lack of concentration

- playing or working under the influence of drugs, alcohol, or strong prescription medicines

If I am injured, what questions should I ask myself?

Set up a mental checklist. If the injury is to your leg, for instance, ask yourself a series of escalating questions: Can I walk? Do I need to be carried? Do I need immediate medical attention? If you structure your problem, you'll be better able to cope with it.

In the event your judgment is impaired, rely on a companion or bystander to evaluate your injury.

What basic supplies should I have in my medicine chest, or even take with me on a lengthy vacation?

That depends on the individual, and what ailments one is prone to. But here are some essentials.

- assorted Band-Aids, adhesives, and gauzes; cotton swabs and balls; scissors and tweezers; Ace bandages and safety pins; ice packs and heat compresses

- over-the-counter pain relievers such as Tylenol, aspirin, and
  ibuprofen; hydrogen peroxide; calamine lotion; antibiotic,
  anti-inflammatory, and antifungal creams; antihistamine pills;
  cough and flu medicines; petroleum jelly and sunscreen

AIDS

Acquired immune deficiency syndrome (AIDS) makes the sufferer
susceptible to a variety of diseases. It is caused by the human im-
munodeficiency virus (HIV), which weakens the body's resistance by
attacking its white blood cells and is spread through infected semen,
vaginal fluid, and blood. AIDS, which is life-threatening, may not appear for years after the HIV presence is detected.

What are some of the illnesses associated with HIV-related infections?

Neurogenic impairment, swelling in the lower extremities, skin lesions, chronic respiratory discomfort, limb and bowel dysfunction—
these are but a small sample.

Left untreated, the symptoms usually worsen, often bringing on
terminal illness.

How common are HIV-related neurological disorders?

They occur frequently, and may even be underreported or masked by
more severe problems. Symptoms include a tingling in the skin and a
partial loss of feeling in the legs or feet. Such impairment limits mobility and can have significant consequences, leading to pneumonia,
blood clots in the venous system, and limb contracture.

How can I reduce the pain in the lower extremities?

Elevating the limbs and moving the joints do much to restore the circulation, thereby reducing swelling and increasing mobility. Various salves and the use of ultraviolet light help heal, or at least control, the skin lesions.

Can I be tested to see if I'm HIV-positive?

Yes, your doctor can give you simple tests. Make sure, however, that you have had AIDS counseling first, so you can cope with the news if it's bad. People in high-risk groups—say, homosexuals who practice unprotected sex or drug users who share needles—should get tested a couple of times a year.

If you test positive, it's essential that you tell those you may have infected. Just as you will need medical help, so will they.

I've heard about all sorts of new drugs that can control AIDS and prolong life. Do they exist?

Hundreds of antibiotic, antiviral, and anticancer drugs are now on the market, and many are being administered to AIDS sufferers, usually in combinations of half a dozen or more and on a complex schedule. They seem to be working, in the sense that they prolong life. But no breakthrough drug currently exists.

Zidovudine, known as AZT, is one common anti-AIDS drug that at least temporarily keeps the virus from propagating. Like many such medications, however, it can have serious side effects, including severe headaches and nausea, and even dementia.

What is meant by the expression "AIDS cocktail"?

This is the description given the multipill regimen that doctors prescribe for those suffering from HIV infections.

The drugs themselves, as well as the combinations in which they are taken, are continually evolving. But the latest "cocktail" calls for an admixture of nucleoside analog drugs, which at least temporarily decrease the amount of viral particles in the blood and increase the number of T cells the body needs to fight infection, and a protease inhibitor, which prevents the breaking down of new proteins the HIV virus is seeking to invade.

Which of the nucleoside analogs are best is a matter of opinion. Certainly AZT had the longest track record. Eventually, however, HIV becomes resistant to AZT, and other nucleoside analogs are added to the "cocktail." Two of these are ddI and ddC.

Common protease inhibitors are ritinovir and indinavir.

The drugs in HIV "cocktails" are continually being adjusted by doctors, depending on how well patients tolerate the mix and how much the medications help them.

What about alternative treatments?

Our immune system seems to benefit if we reduce the stress in our lives, so many of these therapies seek to do just that. Acupuncture, acupressure, heat therapy, biofeedback, and simple meditation can offer relief, but they must be pursued under medical supervision.

What about diet?

Avoid alcohol, caffeine, and sugar—all of which tend to impair white blood cells.

How does the HIV patient's psychological state affect pain perception?

The HIV sufferer has to come to terms with a life-threatening syndrome, and the best way to do so is to reframe the situation in a positive manner. The illness can be seen as a wake-up call, a challenge, a chance to direct one's life toward a new goal.

Such positive thinking raises the pain threshold and gives the patient the moral strength to live each day to the fullest.

How vital is a support network?

It's essential. A support network reinforces the patient's feelings of optimism and hope, and provides a stable, caring environment in which important medical, personal, and financial decisions can be made.

Anal Bleeding

Is anal bleeding always a sign that something is terribly wrong?

Not necessarily. The bleeding may result from hemorrhoids or simply from pushing too hard on the bowels. Hemorrhoids often respond to sitting in warm water several times a day; bowel movements, to the short-term use of suppositories.

Continued bleeding, however, possibly accompanied by nausea or vomiting, may indicate such intestinal problems as colitis, Crohn's disease, or gastroenteritis—all of which require professional treatment.

In worst-case scenarios, such bleeding may also indicate colon cancer or cirrhosis.

Colon cancer requires surgery, called a laparotomy, to excise parts of the bowel. Afterward, if the colon cannot be reconnected to the rectum, a colostomy is performed, allowing waste from the colon to exit the body into an external bag.

Cirrhosis, usually brought on by alcohol abuse, attacks the liver, the largest of the body's organs and a vital part of the digestive and immune systems. Provided the liver is not too far gone, such cirrhosis can be arrested by giving up alcohol. Abstain and live; drink and die.

Aneurysm

An aneurysm is a bulge in an artery, usually the aorta. If the bulge bursts, the patient feels sudden, severe pain and faces a life-threatening situation.

What causes aneurysms, and where do they most often occur?

They usually result from high blood pressure or atherosclerosis, the buildup of fatty deposits in the arteries. Most occur in the abdomen; others, in the chest and neck and even behind the knee.

How are aneurysms found before they actually burst?

Sometimes they're discovered in routine physicals, when the doctor feels a pulsating artery while probing the patient's stomach. Other times they're found through X rays and ultrasound scans.

How are they treated?

Doctors generally recommend surgery if the aneurysm is wider than two inches. The weakened section of the artery is cut away, and the gap is bridged with a synthetic graft.

If the aneurysm is smaller, or if the patient's overall physical condition is poor, doctors often prefer to monitor the situation. Meanwhile, they prescribe medications and dietary modifications to lessen the patient's blood pressure or degree of atherosclerosis.

Anxiety

Is anxiety always focused on a particular event?

Some anxiety states, it is true, may be occasioned by a personal experience, a retained memory, or a specific location. However, many people experience diffuse, or free-floating, bouts of anxiety. These attacks may come on slowly or quickly, apparently without cause. Indeed, if the attack does not have a readily identifiable source, its potency may be all the greater.

Simple causes of anxiety, those on a conscious level, can be handled through meditation and self-examination. But if the causes are myriad and exist on a subconscious level, professional counseling is required.

What is a "panic attack"?

A "panic attack" is the mother of all anxiety states. It involves drastic changes in one's pulse and heart and respiratory rates, and the inability to focus, concentrate, or put thoughts in logical order.

Why does my anxiety make me sick?

Though the sources of anxiety are psychological, beginning with one's thoughts, feelings, and perceptions, the resulting problems are very tangible. Constipation or diarrhea, headache, muscular or joint pain, and, as noted, changes in pulse and heart and respiratory rates are common.

We teach patients how to modify their response to stress. Once they focus their energies not on their plight but on how to handle it, they often find their physical problems receding.

How much professional help is available to treat anxiety?

Doctors, psychologists, and counseling social workers all offer professional help, with both traditional and alternative methods of treatment. Therapies include relaxation techniques, hypnosis, biofeedback, and self-guided imagery.

Some solutions are not even directly linked to the original symptom. Peripheral activities such as caring for a pet, listening to music, and gardening can be beneficial.

When my anxiety increases at night, what techniques will help?

Reduced stimulation during the night often relieves stress symptoms. Self-learned therapies, specifically designed to be used in the home, include music, self-hypnosis, and exercise.

Can I learn to manage my anxiety at the office?

Yes. First, we help the sufferer become fully aware of the circumstances causing the anxiety. Then we suggest such remedies as taking rest breaks, reducing unnecessary noise, and reallocating tasks. In ways large and small, undue pressures can usually be lessened.

How does my daily schedule affect my anxiety?

Time management is a key element to proper scheduling. You must keep appointments, allow enough time for the task at hand, prioritize, and set goals.

Although these principles sound elementary, many people do not follow them and, in essence, bring about their own anxiety. Again, we teach behavior modification, helping patients realize they should keep calendars and date books, improve their written and verbal communication skills, and interrelate with coworkers.

I understand that the human genome will soon be completely mapped out, permitting doctors to treat disease in previously unimaginable detail. But won't these genetic tests cause considerable anxiety in people who learn that they, or their unborn children, *might* come to be affected in the future with severe illnesses?

Genetic testing undoubtedly will create added levels of anxiety, particularly those results that do not give definitive answers but instead indicate only that the patient is at higher risk. One genetic test for breast cancer, for instance, simply tells us the likelihood of the disease occurring, thereby creating worry even though the illness may never strike.

Once again, we ask our patients to adjust their attitudes to anxiety. By focusing their energies not on what might be but on the here and now, they can keep their worries under control.

Appendicitis

The appendix is a tiny tube, only a few inches long, that extends from the large intestine. If it becomes inflamed, it causes severe pain in the lower right abdomen and must be surgically removed as soon as possible.

Why is appendicitis a medical emergency?
Left untreated, the inflamed appendix may rupture, releasing infectious intestinal material into the stomach, resulting in a life-threatening condition called peritonitis.

What causes the problem?
We don't really know. What we do know is that appendicitis is the leading cause of stomach surgery in the United States, that it mostly

strikes people under thirty, and that the appendix itself is a nonessential organ.

Is surgery always called for?

The danger of rupture, and peritonitis, is so great that doctors almost always feel that surgery is the proper treatment.

Patients can be on their feet within hours after the operation, and be discharged in two or three days. Laparoscopic surgery, which lets the surgeon see inside the abdomen through a tiny telescope, ensures a smaller incision and a briefer convalescence than does open abdominal surgery.

What techniques speed healing after the operation?

Acupressure can be helpful. Once a trained therapist shows you the pressure points for the stomach, bladder, and large intestine, you can use the technique yourself, at home, whenever you feel the need.

Arthritis

A painful condition of the joints, arthritis is a very common disorder. Many people suffer from at least mild variations of the disease, encouraging it by a sedentary lifestyle or enduring it as a part of the aging process.

How does arthritis attack the joints?

Understand that the ends of the bones coming together in a joint are cushioned by cartilage, and the joint cavity itself, in and around the cartilage, is sealed by a fluid-filled membrane. If the cartilage degenerates or is torn, or if the membrane becomes inflamed, discomfort results.

What are the principal types of arthritis?

There are two. Rheumatoid arthritis, which is found in women far more frequently than in men, occurs when there is damage to the joint's membrane, resulting in excess fluid in the cavity, swelling, and cartilage deterioration.

Osteoarthritis, or degenerative arthritis, which is found mainly in the elderly, takes place because the joint's cartilage gradually wears down, reducing the cushioning.

A subclassification, infectious arthritis, refers to joint irritation that is a manifestation of some other disease.

Is arthritis a disabling condition?

For the most part, no. While it's true that extreme cases of arthritis can cause loss of hand function, limit movement, and even affect one's ability to walk, the disease more typically involves cyclical bouts of pain. Learning how to mitigate the discomfort is an integral part of the sufferer's therapy.

Are some joints more likely to become arthritic than others?

Not really, although an individual's activities obviously weaken some joints more than others. A middle-aged marathon runner, say, is apt to experience discomfort in the knees.

Arthritis can strike any joint: from neck to shoulders to lower back, from elbows to wrists to fingers, from hips to knees to toes.

Luckily, most people experience arthritis in only a few joints, not in all.

Do behavioral traits affect arthritis?

Placing heavy loads on the joints, whether it is our marathon-runner friend overworking his knees or someone carrying too many pounds, and repetitive pressures of all kinds can certainly exacerbate the inflammation.

Walkers, canes, and other aids are designed to ease these pressures.

Does long-term arthritis sometimes cause deformity?

Yes. Arthritic fluids in the joints may bring on considerable swelling; meanwhile, cartilage erosion may cause misalignment of the limbs.

Does the weather affect arthritis?

It remains a topic of controversy. Nonetheless, many sufferers insist that their pain increases during periods of cold, damp weather, when there are low barometric readings.

What professional remedies exist?

Solutions depend on how badly the joint is damaged, and range from intense physical therapy to injected medications to joint replacement.

If surgery is required, arthroscopy may be possible. This is a procedure less invasive than normal surgery, necessitating less recuperation time.

What home remedies ease the pain of arthritis?

Over-the-counter medications include aspirin, acetaminophen (Tylenol), and the nonsteroidal anti-inflammatory ibuprofen.

Heat also provides relief, whether delivered through a warm bath or compress or through a heating pad.

Friends have told me that glucosamine and chondroitin sulfate, two natural remedies, will help rebuild the worn cartilage between joints. Is this true?

Glucosamine is made from crushed crab shells and chondroitin sulfate from the windpipes of cows. The theory is that their molecular structure resembles cartilage molecules and that over time the ingestion of these substances will restore worn cartilage. The two remedies certainly have their believers. Sales totaled some $700 million in 1999, an increase of 60 percent over 1998. Even McNeil Consumer Healthcare, the maker of Tylenol and Motrin, is getting into the business, offering glucosamine under the name Aflexa.

The *Journal of the American Medical Association* has given the products mixed reviews. One article stated that while the benefits may have been exaggerated, the substances probably offered "some degree of efficacy." Dr. Tim McAlindon, assistant professor of medicine at the Boston University School of Medicine's Arthritis Center and the lead author of the *JAMA* piece, stated that "they might work, but people need to be apprised of the fact that there is still a possibility that time will show they don't work."

Because the products are a dietary supplement, they aren't treated as drugs by the Food and Drug Administration, and therefore control over the ingredients is limited. In this regard, an independent testing firm found that half of the chrondroitin sulfate brands didn't contain as much of the substance as promised. (Chondroitin sulfate is four times as expensive to manufacture as glucosamine.) Most manufacturers recommend a combination of 500 mg of glucosamine and 400 mg of chondroitin sulfate taken three times a day.

People with shellfish allergies, obviously, should avoid the supplements, as should those with diabetes or on blood-thinning medications. That's because glucosamine increases blood-sugar levels, and chondroitin sulfate is chemically similar to the blood thinners heparin and warfarin.

I understand that rheumatoid arthritis is commonly treated with nonsteroidal anti-inflammatory drugs (NSAIDs). Can you recommend one such medication above the rest?

No one NSAID has ever been shown to be more efficacious or to produce fewer side effects than any other. This means that if one NSAID isn't easing your pain, or indeed is causing you additional discomfort, your physician will prescribe another. It's a trial-and-error approach to pain management, and it's perfectly legitimate. Highly rated NSAIDs include Naprosyn, Relafen, Daypro, Motrin, Aleve, and Ansaid.

What can you tell me about scorpion venom being used to treat arthritis and lupus?

One study at the University of California at Irvine has developed a synthetic chemical, tram-34, that was inspired by the way scorpion poison affects the cells of its victims. The venom, which is usually not fatal, activates the body's immune response system. But tram-34 conversely suppresses T cells, part of the body's defense system against foreign intruders, without harming the production of enzymes and other important cell functions.

Tram-34 is still in the experimental stage.

What are the cutting-edge developments in the creation of new bone and cartilage to ease the pain of arthritis?

Researchers at the University of California's graduate bioengineering group have reported changing human skin, at least at the laboratory level, into substantial amounts of bone and cartilage. Within the dermis, the skin's middle layer, are a multitude of so-called fibroblasts. These are the cells that Dr. Rajendra Bhatnagar, head of the group, has successfully converted into new tissue. He reported generating from a snip of skin no more than a few cubic millimeters in volume enough tissue to fill a hole in bone or cartilage many hundreds of times that size.

Dr. Bhatnagar hopes that fibroblast technology can be developed to the point where it eliminates the need for the half a million hip and knee replacements that are performed each year. "Sounds like science fiction, doesn't it?" he remarked. "But that's what we do."

Athletic Injuries

What is the primary cause of sports injuries?
The chief culprit is sudden or repetitive stress on the bones or on the tissues around the bones (the muscles, tendons, cartilage, and ligaments), resulting in fractures, dislocations, tears, or bruises.

How do the various tissues differ in their functions?
- Muscles contract and react, facilitating bone movement.

- Tendons connect the muscles to the bones.

- Cartilage, found mostly in the joints, cushions the bones where they meet.

- Ligaments connect one bone to another.

Where in the body do most bone and tissue injuries occur?
Just about anywhere. Starting from the top: collarbone, shoulder, and rotator cuff; lower back; elbow, wrist, and hand; quadriceps, hamstring, and knee; shin, ankle, and foot.

Collarbones are commonly fractured, and shoulders dislocated or separated because of torn ligaments, in contact sports. Rotator cuff injuries, to the tendons in the muscles behind the shoulder, result from forceful, repetitive movements, such as pitching a baseball.

Lower back strains, in the muscles surrounding the spine, are brought on by violent twists and turns.

Elbow ligaments likewise are damaged by twisting movements, such as rotating the forearm to put spin on a tennis ball. Wrist and finger problems result from falls and collisions.

Groin pulls are painful tears in the muscle between the leg and the pubic bone. Tendinitis in the knee comes from too much jumping, while sharp blows to the quadriceps muscle above the knee produce near paralyzing bruises. Straining the hamstrings, the tendons behind the knee, is similarly disabling.

Overusing the muscles in the lower legs, perhaps from excessive running or jogging, all but guarantees shin splints, Achilles tendon damage, heel pain, or even stress fractures.

Generally speaking, how are these conditions treated?

X rays find the more obvious fractures and dislocations, but bone scans may be needed to locate stress fractures. Magnetic resonance imaging (MRI) is the tool of choice in pinpointing muscle, tendon, and ligament problems.

Medications include painkillers ranging from aspirin to codeine, anti-inflammatories, and corticosteroids. Massage can also be beneficial.

What does the acronym RICE mean?

It signifies the standard treatment for tissue damage: rest, ice, compression, and elevation.

What should I know about concussions?

They're not bruises to the brain, as popular wisdom regards them. Indeed, no physical swelling or bleeding usually occurs. Concussions are caused by blows to the head that create chemical imbalances. Brain cells fire off chemicals all at once, overwhelming receptors linked to learning and memory. Symptoms include confusion, nausea, blurred vision, even loss of consciousness. In severe cases, recovery can take a considerable time.

What are these chemicals you speak of?

They're calcium, potassium, and sodium ions, and they contract the arteries and make it difficult for nutrients to reach the injured brain cells. These damaged cells need substantial amounts of glucose, but the high demand cannot be met because of the narrowed arteries. This mismatch creates a metabolic crisis, particularly during the first day or so after the injury.

If I have one concussion, am I likely to get more?

Neurologists say that once a person suffers one concussion, he or she is four times more likely to get another. Moreover, with each succeeding concussion it takes less of a blow to set off the injury and more time to heal.

Does this mean that a man or woman who has suffered a concussion should give up contact sports?

Not necessarily. Each case has to be considered individually. But the concussion must be allowed sufficient time to heal—a period that ranges from days to weeks. Resuming a contact sport too soon after suffering this type of injury is not prudent.

Do you have any other tips?

- Do some easy warm-ups before extending yourself. Stretching exercises loosen the tendons and ligaments; jogging in place accelerates blood flow, making the muscles more pliable.

- If you're over thirty, give up contact sports.

You mention doing warm-ups. How much warming up and stretching is necessary?

A recent report in *The Physician and Sportsmedicine* dispels a good many myths on this subject:

- Stretching before exercise apparently does not decrease the risk of injury but does reduce pain from stiffness.

- Warming up—doing light exercises—does not increase the range of motion but does reduce the chance of injury, probably by raising the temperature of the muscle tissue.

- "Bounce" stretching—repeatedly doing brief stretches—can increase stiffness and actually be harmful.

- One fifteen-to-thirty-second continuous stretch is usually enough for most muscle groups.

- Using heat or cold on a muscle makes the stretching more effective.

- Warming up and stretching programs should be tailored to the individual, depending upon his or her history of injuries.

Back Pain (lower)

Next to the common cold, lower back pain is probably the biggest reason people miss a day's work. The labor cost of these absences is enormous, and companies large and small are increasingly emphasizing preventive and self-help techniques in their medical insurance coverage.

What causes lower back pain?

Here we're talking about pain in the lumbar vertebrae region. The causes include arthritis, muscle strain, slipped discs, small congenital malformations of the spine, and torn ligaments.

The vertebrae have differing anatomical structures, each relating to one another depending on bodily movement. If arthritis sets in, for instance, it interferes with this delicate relationship, causing pain and limiting movement. Diagnosing precisely where the pain is among the vertebrae can be difficult.

What do back braces accomplish?

Back braces, or lumbar supports, do not make the spine more capable of movement but rather give the lower back more support and ensure better posture.

The trade-off, or downside, is that prolonged use of braces may weaken the natural support of the abdominal muscles. These muscles are essential to maintaining healthful posture.

Braces are best used on a temporary basis, to remind people that they may be overdoing a particular bodily movement. In this sense, they give people a psychological, as well as a physical, parameter to control their exertions.

What is the role of exercise in lower back pain?

Exercise stimulates the lumbar area and the abdominals and enhances posture. Passive therapies, such as massage and electrical stimulation, are no substitute for vigorous, but controlled, physical activity.

Here are two simple exercises, not only to forestall lower back problems but to relieve existing pain:

1. Lie on your back on the floor, arms straight along your sides. Take a deep breath, then exhale, simultaneously contracting your abdominals and pressing your lower back against the floor. You may have to raise your knees slightly while pushing down your back. Do ten repetitions, gradually increasing to twenty-five.

2. Lie on your back on the floor, feet together, knees bent at a forty-five-degree angle, hands clasped behind your neck. Take a deep breath, then exhale, simultaneously raising your back and head a few inches from the floor. Your weight should be supported by your feet and abdominals, *not* by your back and neck. Hold the position for a second or two, then slowly lower your back and head to the floor. Do ten reps, building up to twenty-five.

When should I rest and when should I exercise?

Rest is important during the acute stage of pain, when the nerve is swollen or irritated. Then the sufferer can be taught, through proper medical guidance, to develop an internal warning system—a thermostat, so to speak. When the indicators go up, rest; when they go down, exercise. One of the basic aims of exercise therapy is to make patients knowledgeable about their condition, helping them attain independence.

Understand that lumbar pain often results when the nerve chafes within the vertebra, either because the nerve is swollen or because the opening is too narrow. Medical care calls either for reducing the swelling—perhaps using some type of cortisone injection—or for increasing the size of the opening, perhaps by alternating hot and cold therapies to relax the surrounding muscles.

What diagnostic procedures should I expect?

For starters, every patient needs an X ray. Many people talk to friends and think the treatments that worked for their friends will work for them. The fallacy here is that no two back pains have the same origin.

CAT scans and MRIs, computerized tests, show the anatomy of the spine in greater detail than X rays: CAT scans are X-ray-based: MRIs are generated by a magnetic field. PET scans, which are metabolic-based, are also available, but their efficacy in the lumbar area in still under debate.

EMGs, electrode studies using fine needles and mild electrical currents, analyze neural impulses. Thermography calls for infrared cameras to register temperature variations, producing images of abnormal tissue growth.

Depending on the complexity of the problem, many or most of these studies may be required before doctors, correlating the results, can make a proper diagnosis.

When should I seek professional help for lower back pain?

We suggest the "right-angle," or ninety-degree, criterion—meaning you should see a doctor as soon as you experience significant pain but are still upright. *Don't* wait for the "horizontal," or 180-degree, stage, when you're flat on your back. Toughing it out is foolish.

How do work and home environments affect my condition?

It's the small, accumulative activities occurring throughout the day that determine the amount of stress on the lower back. Using the wrong office and household furnishings and equipment can compound the problem.

Ergonomics experts are redesigning furnishings and equipment to reduce such stress, and we have learned a great deal from them. An office worker sitting on a chair, for instance, will tell you she is comfortable. But if experts place electrodes on her lower back, the readings show that her vertebrae are under pressure.

So when we talk to pain sufferers, we want to know what kind of chair they sit in or bed they sleep on or computer keyboard they use. It's part of getting to know, and treat, the whole patient.

What is fibromyalgia?

It's a chronic disease characterized by musculoskeletal pain, often in the back area, but it's neither an inflammatory condition nor a degenerative ailment. Skeptics have concluded that the problem exists only in the victim's mind. But as we keep stressing, this criticism misses the point. The victim's pain is real, and must be treated.

Fibromyalgia is often compared to spinal disc degeneracy, osteoporosis, or even Lyme disease. Many of its victims suffer from other ailments that may be psychological in origin—chronic fatigue syndrome, headaches, or irritable bowel syndrome.

Treatment calls for getting enough sleep, relieving stress, avoiding exposure to dampness and cold, and keeping the muscle joints and tendons flexible. Leg stretches can be done with a chair from a standing position; back stretches, with a towel from a sitting position.

For leg stretches: (1) Stand with your feet moderately apart, leaning forward, behind a straight-back chair; (2) bend your upper torso, keeping your knees straight, until you feel tension in your leg muscles, then relax; (3) do ten reps, gradually building up to twenty-five.

For back stretches: (1) Sit on the floor, knees straight, looping a towel around your feet; (2) gently pull your torso forward until you feel tension in your back muscles, then relax; (3) do ten reps, gradually building up to twenty-five.

Body Lumps

Regularly examining your body for lumps or protrusions on or beneath the skin may help you spot problems before they become serious.

What are some trouble spots?

- Swollen lymph nodes, particularly in the neck or armpits, can be a sign of lymphoma or mononucleosis.

- Lumps in a woman's breasts can indicate cancer, as can lumps in a man's testicles.

- Small growths on the skin's surface, especially if they change color, can be cancerous.

- Lumps in the groin can indicate a hernia.

What should I do if I find something?

See your doctor immediately.

Bone Fractures

Why does breaking a bone hurt so much?

The nerve receptors in bones are extremely sensitive. They receive and transmit a pain deeper and longer-lasting than the receptors in soft tissue.

Why do extremities swell after a bone fracture?

The edema, or swelling, is caused by the accumulation of fluids near the site of the fracture. Initially, simple remedies such as cooling the area with ice packs or elevating the extremity can reduce the discomfort.

What is the role of the cast in healing fractures?

For a bone to heal, the broken elements must be immobilized while touching each other. A cast or brace accomplishes this. Once the healing phase is completed, the cast is removed and the rehabilitation begins.

What is the recovery scenario in bone-fracture cases?

Early on, the pain is most intense.

Then the decision is made, depending on the complexity of the break, to treat the fracture either surgically or nonsurgically. In the former case, metal hardware is used to line up the segments. Sometimes bone grafting is also done to promote the healing.

Nonsurgical correction calls for a cast. Traction may also be used.

As the bone heals, the limb experiences atrophy, or weakness, because of disuse. The skin also dries out, because of the cast and other dressings. The pain and discomfort, though much relieved, continue.

What does it mean for a bone to "knit"?

This is a colloquial expression used to describe the healing phase of bone fractures. Once a break occurs, each end of the bone responds by laying down new bone, or "knitting." This bone is called callous formation.

Bone healing, or "knitting," occurs in response to both traumatic fractures and surgically created fractures (which allow the success of bone grafting).

Are some of us more likely than others to have fractures?

Yes. The bone health of the individual determines the level of future risk. People with osteoporosis, for instance, are more vulnerable to fracture, as are the nutritionally deprived and those with underlying metabolic diseases.

Luckily, proper drug treatment can improve bone strength, or at least arrest its decay.

Can diet contribute to the likelihood of bone fractures?

Perhaps. At least one study suggests that women who habitually drink cola are five times more likely to have fractures as those who do not. Some believe that the phosphoric acid in cola drinks is the culprit, because it may adversely affect calcium metabolism and bone mass.

Others believe that long-term cola drinking, particularly when begun at an early age, replaces the milk drinking that young people, both male and female, need to develop strong bones.

How does osteoporosis affect my health?

Besides increasing the chance of major fractures, osteoporosis increases the likelihood of multiple hairline breaks. These fractures can lead to a compression of the spine, forcing sufferers into a stooped posture.

This disforming posture causes extreme discomfort, not only in the back but also, because of the pressure, on the lungs and intestines.

Bone Spurs

What are bone spurs?
They're abnormal growths at the end of bones, often occurring in the joints. Because they're not cushioned by cartilage, they tend to rub against adjacent bone and tissue, causing considerable pain.

What causes them?
Sometimes they're part of the aging process; sometimes they're brought on by repetitive stress.

Where are the spurs most often found?
In the neck and back. What happens is that the discs, the cushions between the vertebrae, weaken and bulge outward, irritating the spinal nerves.

The pain can remain centered in the neck and back, or it can radiate to the buttocks and thighs, a condition called sciatica.

I've heard people complain of bone spurs in the heels of their feet. What causes the pain there?
The spurs grow out of the base of the heel, inflaming the connective tissue, or plantar fascia, between the heel and toes.

How are spurs treated?
Usually through painkillers and anti-inflammatory drugs, the latter taken orally or injected directly into the affected area. Bed rest is

needed for disc problems, but just laying off running or jogging, plus placing a circular foam pad over the irritation, alleviates heel spurs.

Surgery is recommended only if the pain is unremitting, or complicating factors worsen the condition.

Burns

Burns to the skin, a bodily organ replete with nerve endings and blood vessels, range from first degree burns (redness) to second degree (blistering) to third degree (scorched down to the blood vessels) to fourth degree (scorched to the bone).

What is the skin's function?

The skin is multilayered, from epidermis to dermis to fat, and each layer performs an assigned task. "Dead cells" on the surface, for instance, protect us from sunlight's ultraviolet rays and prevent the loss of excess fluid. Our pores allow us to sweat, thereby stabilizing bodily temperatures. Lower skin layers are metabolically active, promoting the healing process after such injuries as burns and cuts. Finally, the fat layer provides insulation against extremes of temperature.

Why do burns in certain parts of the body hurt more than in others?

Burns are more painful in those areas with the greatest number of nerve endings, such as the face or fingers, or in those places where the skin must be particularly elastic, such as the shoulder, elbow, and knee joints.

What are the long-term consequences of severe burns?

The deeper the burn, the greater the incidence of shock, loss of healing fluids, length of recuperation, and risk of scarring and unsightly growths.

How do burns heal?

First-degree burns usually can be treated with creams that preserve and enhance the skin's water content and have an analgesic additive. Second-degree burns require extra care to prevent infection in the blistered skin, which might cause scarring.

With third- and fourth-degree burns, skin actually is destroyed, and usually is replaced by scar tissue. The larger the damaged area, the more disabling the condition. Surgically removing the growth, and grafting healthy skin over the injury, often is necessary.

Is butter good for a burn?

Putting butter or oil on a burn is not particularly effective. Nor is using alcohol or menthol, irritants that only accentuate the problem. Nor is treating the burn with water, since by itself water lacks the electrolytes needed to stimulate the flow of healing molecules.

Medicated creams, specially compounded to speed the rehydration process, are the preferred remedy.

Why do some burns heal with scars?

Deeper burns damage the skin's regenerating layers, preventing its regrowth. Replacing it is scar tissue, which lacks healthy skin's intricate structure and active metabolism.

What are some home remedies for simple burns?

Aloe is an excellent natural remedy, and it can be applied as a lotion, cream, gel, or even directly in plant form. Soothing salves, such as cold cream, also are beneficial.

In general, covering an open burn eases the pain experienced on exposure to air. However, the choice of dressing is important. Bandages and Band-Aids that do not "stick" to the healing area are essential.

What is the recovery schedule for severe burns?

Recovery time depends, to a great extent, on how extensively the skin is damaged, and how deeply it is penetrated. Complicating the picture is the location of the burn, particularly if it crosses a joint.

Even after healing occurs, however, the patient may face long-term problems: the emotional pain of dealing with scars, the debilitating effect of repeated surgery, the tedium of immobilization. Rehabilitation can be a drawn-out process.

Bursitis

A bursa is a fluid-filled sac or cushion within the soft tissue around a joint. Its job is to ensure the proper movement of the joint and to absorb shocks. When this sac becomes inflamed, bursitis results.

What are the symptoms of bursitis?

Joint pain, tenderness, and limited range of motion.

What makes a bursa painful?

The fluid-filled bursa is housed in a limited space. When inflammation occurs, fluids and toxins accumulate in the sac, making it swell. The pain results from both pressure on the sac and compression on the joint. It's a double-edged whammy.

What exacerbates bursitis?

Usually repeated abuse of the joints, through either violent movements or excessive strain.

What part does heat play in relieving the symptoms?

In mild cases, we prescribe therapeutic heat to improve circulation,
clear toxins, and reduce fluid accumulation. Together with aspirin,
gentle massage, and elevation of the joint, this generally brings relief.

When do you drain a bursa?

We drain in more extreme cases, partially to ease the patient's discomfort more quickly. But aspiration, or fluid removal using a sterile
needle, also helps us treat the problem. The fluid itself, which can be
analyzed to detect various joint conditions, becomes a significant diagnostic tool. (If fluid reaccumulates, a series of aspirations may be
needed.)

Conversely, medications such as corticosteroids may be injected
directly into the joints to lessen inflammation and pain. (Caution:
Such steroid injections should not be overdone, lest they cause long-
term harm.)

What is adhesive capsulitis?

This condition occurs when the fibrous surface of the bursa itself
adheres to the joint, with resulting irritation. To counteract the "stick-
ing" effect, we use more penetrating forms of heat and more intense
forms of physical therapy.

What joints are commonly affected by bursitis?

The shoulder, elbow, hip, and knee.

Shoulder, elbow, and knee problems may be relieved by protective pads, and hip and knee conditions by canes, crutches, and walkers, in addition to the options already described.

What are the most common medications?

Nonsteroidal anti-inflammatory drugs (NSAIDs), including aspirin, ibuprofen, Motrin, Advil, and other nonnarcotic analgesics, as well as steroids.

What are reflex sympathetic dystrophy (RSD) and shoulder-hand syndrome?

Both are sometimes confused with bursitis, but they can be more serious.

RSD is a neurological type of pain that is accompanied by swelling and stiffening. Treatment can call for a surgical nerve block.

Shoulder-hand syndrome is damage to the shoulder's rotator cuff, with attendant pain and swelling. Therapy initially calls for rest and strengthening exercises but can necessitate surgery.

Cancer Pain

We use the term *cancer* to describe scores of diseases in all parts of the body, from the bloodstream to the organs, from muscle to bone. Our cells somehow multiply out of control, creating tumors, and sometimes these tumors are malignant.

The pain that results from cancer can be both acute and chronic, and alleviating it demands cutting-edge medical skill.

What are the principal treatments for cancer?

Surgery, radiation, and chemotherapy.

Why do cancer sufferers seek alternative solutions to their pain?

One reason is that cancer pain can be so intense that failure with traditional methods understandably drives desperate sufferers to alternative therapies.

Another reason is that many traditional doctors are not adequately treating the pain. The *Journal of the American Medical Association* reports that 90 percent of those suffering severe discomfort could have been helped through sedation but were not.

Why? In part because many states, unduly fearful that doctors' offices will be used to distribute drugs illegally, restrict the number of painkillers a doctor can prescribe for a single patient.

But also in part because some doctors, says the *Wall Street Journal*, "don't want to look like pushers." Continues the *Journal*: "But when administered properly, painkillers can actually make patients more alert."

Dr. Charles Cleeland of the Anderson Cancer Center, author of the *JAMA* editorial, maintains that some doctors "think it is highly risky to give an elderly patient opiates when it really is the opposite. Elderly patients can tolerate and need the medicine."

Warns Dr. Cleeland: "Doctors continue to have a poor sense of how many patients have pain." We agree. Sufferers should let their doctors know, long and loud, when they are hurting.

What is touch therapy?

This alternative technique, admittedly controversial, involves the use of gentle touch, or even near touch, to "draw off" the sufferer's pain. One part massage, one part compassion, the therapy strives to relieve the tension compounding the patient's discomfort.

Why is TENS often used in treating cancer pain?

TENS, short for transcutaneous electrical nerve stimulation, involves a portable electronic device that can easily be used at home. It passes a mild electrical current through surface electrodes and eases the sensation of pain. It does not pierce the skin or deliver heat or chemicals. It probably encourages the body to produce additional endorphins.

Because TENS can be used any hour of the day or night, it is ideal for treating cancer pain. One caution: TENS should not be used by people with electronic implants.

What should I know about breast cancer?

Don't go into denial. If you think you may have a tumor, seek treatment immediately. Fear of a possible mastectomy is understandable, but fear of death should be your prime consideration.

Fifty thousand American women die of breast cancer each year, and it kills with greater regularity the longer treatment is delayed. At stage one, the least serious level when cancer is confined to the breast, the five-year survival rate is 85 percent. At stage four, when it is widespread, the rate is 20 percent.

Yet at least one-third of women who discover a lump in their breasts delay seeing a doctor for at least three months. Don't be one of them.

I have heard that the symptoms of oral cancer frequently are overlooked. What are they?

They include sores on the lip or in the mouth or throat, as well as red or white spots on the gums, tongue, or lining of the mouth. Also, unusual bleeding or numbness in the mouth, persistent sore throats, or swelling in the jaw.

Can alternative treatments for cancer be effective?

Possibly, particularly if they are applied in tandem with conventional treatments. While radiation, chemotherapy, and surgery remain proven techniques for curing or at least arresting the disease, there is every reason to address the emotional and spiritual needs of the patient. The whole man or woman should be cared for, not just the person's body. Many mainstream oncologists realize this, complementing traditional procedures with diet and exercise programs as well as meditation.

The case can be made, although it cannot be proved, that sufferers who ignore their emotional and spiritual needs are contributing to their malaise.

Of course, we use a sophisticated array of sedatives to mitigate the pain. Equally important, however, is the emotional buttress we can offer.

We had a friend dying of prostate cancer. One day while visiting him, we saw that he had soiled his sheets. Though at first he protested, we cleaned him and freshened his bed. Then we cried and hugged. We had helped our friend make it through another day.

What specifically are the best drugs for treating cancer?

That question can only be answered with many qualifications. The list of medications is long and ever changing. Each patient, and his or her tolerance of pain and a drug's side effects, is different. Each type of cancer requires special consideration.

We could tell you that brain cancer is treated with vincristine, but this is not written in stone. We are not talking about taking an aspirin, we are talking about prescribing a drug in a life-or-death situation. Without knowing the details of a particular case, we would be remiss to say that someone's brain cancer would be best treated with vincristine.

The happy news is that the number of beneficial drugs is ever increasing: cyclophosphamide for Ewing's sarcoma, chlorambucil for leukemia, cisplatin for ovarian cancer—these are but a few. But other drugs may be more suitable for your condition. Only your oncologist can truly advise you.

Then what can you tell me about the latest developments in cancer drugs—at least in general terms?

The newest approach is called molecular targeting, and it takes its name from the use of experimental drugs that strike selectively at cancerous cells to disrupt their activities.

Monoclonal antibodies, for instance, are proteins designed to detect and bind to other proteins that are present in cancer cells, thwarting the cancer's ability to grow. Other drugs, known as angiogenesis inhibitors, stymie the growth of new blood vessels, thereby depriving malignant cells of oxygen and nourishment.

Someone told me that too much calcium in the diet is a leading cause of prostate cancer. Is this true?

A 1998 study in the journal *Cancer Research* reported on the calcium intake, from both dairy products and supplements, of 50,000 men. Those who ingested more calcium, rather than less, were four to eight times at higher risk for the most aggressive form of prostate cancer. Walter Willett, professor and chairman of the Department of Nutrition at the Harvard School of Public Health and coauthor of the study, stated: "I don't think it's the final word, but it needs looking at."

The purchase of calcium supplements totals some $700 million yearly. That figure doesn't include dairy products enriched with calcium; in 1999 marketers introduced 234 such products, four times the number introduced four years earlier.

A second study, this one appearing in 1996 in *Nutrition Review,*

noted that 10 percent of U.S. adults exceed the recommended intake
of calcium and suggested that the influx of fortified products was
responsible. The National Academy of Science warns that no more
than 2,500 mg of calcium should be consumed daily.

Again, we repeat one of our mantras: moderation in all things.

Can viruses be used to kill cancer cells?

Research in this area is currently being pursued, but the results, while
promising, have not been proved. One such form of cancer treatment
involves a virus known as ONYX-015, which has been used in a Phase
II clinical trial—meaning that only a small number of patients were
involved. The virus, which can grow only in cancerous cells, shrank
tumors in the head or neck of almost two-thirds of those treated by
some 50 percent.

This breakthrough was all the more encouraging because most
of the patients had previously failed to respond to surgery or radiation
and were considered incurable. Dr. Faldo R. Khuri of the University
of Texas's M. D. Anderson Cancer Center in Houston, speaking for
himself and the other doctors involved in the trial, said he was "cau-
tiously optimistic" and was looking forward to a larger test. "Many
things look wonderful in Phase Two but not in Phase Three," he ex-
plained.

Why is cancer pain so intense?

Because the pain often consists of so many components. Metastasis,
for instance, can transmit the pain from the original site to other parts
of the body, usually through the blood vessels or lymphatics. Nerves
can become inflamed, damaging surrounding muscles and tissue. The
pain experience in cancer encompasses the disease itself, the effects
of bodily erosion, the difficulties associated with compressing the tumor, the accumulation of fluids and toxins, and diverse other factors.

We must also recognize that the treatment itself may augment the pain. Certain forms of radiation and chemotherapy can cause nausea, vomiting, and overall bodily weakness. The immune system can be compromised, with attendant weight loss, rashes, and ulcers. Finally, the possibility exists that in killing the cancer cells, we destroy adjacent normal cells—winning the battle but losing the war.

The fight against cancer is, admittedly, grim business.

How important are family and friends in helping the patient manage cancer pain?

They play a vital role. Even in the best of times, we live to the fullest and are happiest only in the company of those closest to us. In the worst of times, we need their support all the more.

Family and friends, acting selflessly, can bathe sufferers in their love, washing away negative feelings exacerbating their discomfort.

How do I deal with the depression associated with cancer?

Isolation, hopelessness, physical loss, financial pressures, pain associated with ongoing treatment, feelings of failure associated with recurring disease—any or all of these factors drastically lower one's spirits. We tell our cancer patients that such depression is normal. To overcome their depression, they must acknowledge it.

In the terminal stages of the disease, can cancer patients still be offered hope?

Sadly, only in a sense. At some point patients realize that their lives are slipping away. But usually it is impossible for them, emotionally, to accept the fact. The best all of us can do is provide a support system, helping the patients cope with their suffering on a daily, even hourly, basis.

Carpal Tunnel Syndrome (CTS)

The carpal tunnel is an area in the hand surrounded by connective tissue, or fascia. One of the elements within the tunnel is the median nerve. When this nerve is pinched, pain or a pins-and-needles feeling results. Typically, the sensation occurs in the wrists, hands, and middle fingers.

What activities aggravate carpal tunnel syndrome?

Repetitive activities involving the hand and wrist, such as typing on a computer keyboard or hitting a golf or tennis ball, are thought by many to trigger the syndrome, but this theory has not yet been proved and, in any event, does not eliminate other causes.

Blows to the median nerve, tumors or growths that compress the tunnel, or even the edema in joints that is associated with pregnancy can induce similar pain.

Middle-aged women, particularly those with a weight problem, are especially prone to incur CTS.

Is there a test that will indicate whether the cause of my pain is CTS?

Your doctor may give you the "reverse prayer" test, asking you to place your hands back-to-back, fingernails touching. If a tingling sensation results, the problem has been identified.

How do I relieve the pain?

Mild discomfort is eased by cold compresses, splints to keep the wrists from bending while sleeping, or wrist supports during the workday.

Simple exercises to strengthen wrist and forearm muscles include vigorously opening and closing your fists ten times, resting, then repeating the drill several times. Squeezing a hand-grip device is even more beneficial.

More severe pain requires anti-inflammatory medications, perhaps anti-inflammatory injections into the tunnel, diuretics to reduce the swelling in the soft tissue, or long-term rest and recuperation.

Cataracts and Glaucoma

What are cataracts?

Cataracts occur when the eye's pupil, or lens, ordinarily clear and black, gradually begins to cloud. The condition, while painless, keeps light from reaching the retina, resulting in blurred vision. Left untreated, cataracts can cause blindness.

Who gets them?

Three-quarters of all cataracts are the result of aging, usually in people over seventy. Too much sunlight may hasten the onset of the problem.

Are they difficult to cure?

Not if patients avail themselves of the latest surgical techniques. Some half a million such operations are performed in the United States yearly, the overwhelming number successfully.

How are they diagnosed?

Doctors can find cataracts during routine examinations just by shining a light on the pupil. Later, an ophthalmologist, using a special instrument called a slit lamp, can pinpoint their exact location and level of opacity.

Cataracts, in their early stages at least, need not be removed immediately. But when they worsen, surgery is necessary.

What does treatment consist of?

The operation, done on an outpatient basis under local anesthesia, involves removing the clouded lens and replacing it with a clear plastic implant.

One eye is done at a time, with the patient wearing eyeglasses for several weeks afterward, until completely healed.

What is glaucoma?

The eye is bathed by a thin fluid, called the aqueous humor, that runs over the lens, iris, and cornea and drains from the eye through an outflow channel. If the drainage is blocked, pressure increases on the optic nerve, resulting in pain, "blind spots," and tunnel vision.

Unless it is relieved, the pressure can cause blindness.

How does chronic glaucoma differ from acute glaucoma?

Chronic, or open-angle, glaucoma is by far the most prevalent, causing nine out of every ten cases. It usually affects both eyes at once and occurs gradually, when fluid does not drain fast enough through the outflow channels. Acute, or closed-angle, glaucoma most often affects a single eye and strikes suddenly, when the iris pushes into the cornea, blocking one of the channels.

Who are at risk?

Chronic glaucoma usually develops as we get older, especially among diabetics and the nearsighted. Acute glaucoma can strike at any age and may have a genetic cause.

How are the conditions treated?

Chronic glaucoma is the less serious of the two, and the idea is to either decrease the amount of fluid in the eye or increase drainage.

Various drops, including beta-blockers, pilocarpine, and epinephrine, usually do one or the other.

Acute glaucoma, with the iris itself causing the blockage, presents a different problem. The same medicated drops are used to relieve the condition, but ultimately laser surgery may be employed.

Does diet affect glaucoma?

Perhaps. Some experts feel that vitamin C plays a key role in lowering pressure within the eye. Foods high in this vitamin include oranges, grapefruits, broccoli, and cauliflower.

Cerebral Palsy

This condition in the central nervous system is usually caused by brain damage at or before birth and is marked by spasms and muscular impairment. It sometimes also causes cognitive disorders, such as speech and learning difficulties. Cerebral palsy, which does not become evident until eighteen months of age, affects perhaps one out of every thousand infants but is ten times more common in premature births.

Why do children and adults affected by cerebral palsy appear to be in such discomfort?

Muscular spasms bring on limb contracture and habitual bad posture, creating problems in walking, keeping one's balance, even sitting or lying flat. Ordinary tasks such as dressing and eating become laborious.

How many such sufferers develop epilepsy?

Perhaps a quarter develop severe neurological seizures, commonly called epilepsy.

How can cerebral palsy be managed?

The spasms can be reduced through anticonvulsant medications, and limited mobility in the joints can be relieved through physical therapy and maintenance exercises.

In advanced cases, surgery may be necessary to loosen tightened muscles and tendons.

What about speech and learning problems?

Speech therapy can greatly improve communication skills.

Learning problems are another matter. While many children with cerebral palsy attend regular schools and grow up normally, as many as 60 percent have below-average intelligence and require lifetime assistance.

Chest Pain (heartburn and panic attacks, angina and atherosclerosis, heart attack, blood clots)

Heartburn, which starts out in the abdomen, produces a burning sensation in the chest, especially after meals. Antacids such as Zantac and Pepcid generally relieve the symptoms within minutes. Panic attacks can also produce chest pain. The attacks are caused by stress and can be handled by learning how to cope with stress or how to avoid it. Angina and atherosclerosis, heart attacks, and pulmonary embolisms are more serious matters.

What is angina, and how does it differ from a heart attack?

Angina is the severe but temporary pain felt when the coronary arteries are partially blocked and the brain does not get enough oxygen. As such, it is an early warning that you are at risk for a life-threatening heart attack.

Where is the pain felt?

Generally in the chest, but also in the abdomen, arms, shoulders, neck, or jaw.

What is the primary cause of angina, and what can be done about it?

Fatty deposits in the arteries, a condition called atherosclerosis, are the chief culprits. Therapy initially calls for such medications as beta-blockers, nitrates, and calcium blockers, but, for the long haul, patients must restructure their lifestyle—losing weight, exercising, and giving up fatty foods and tobacco.

In some instances, surgery may be needed.

If angina pain comes and goes, can it be confused with heartburn?

It's true that an electrocardiogram (ECG) may not detect angina, but ultrasound scans and radionuclide imaging are quite reliable. If any doubt exists, doctors may order an angiography, injecting a harmless dye into the arteries to make the pictures easier to read.

Can you tell me more about atherosclerosis, and how it's treated?

Atherosclerosis, which like angina is tied closely to diet and a lack of exercise, occurs when fatty deposits in the arteries slowly calcify and turn to plaque, clogging the flow of blood.

Perhaps the most effective way to treat this condition is a procedure called angioplasty. A catheter—a slim, flexible tube with a deflated balloon at the tip—is threaded into the artery until it is under the plaque. Once the balloon is inflated, the blockage is cleared.

A variation on this procedure uses a stent, an expandable piece of wire mesh, instead of a balloon. The idea is that the metal stent will be more durable than the balloon and keep the passage open longer.

I've heard that chelation therapy will help atherosclerosis. What is it, and does it work?

Chelation therapy, which may require dozens of sessions, involves injecting an anticalcium agent into the arteries that, chelation's supporters say, dissolves plaque.

The technique's effectiveness is still open to question, in the sense that no definitive scientific study yet supports the claim.

Do people experience sporadic pain, as in angina, in the days before a full-fledged heart attack?

Perhaps two-thirds have chest pain and allied symptoms, but a significant number have no warning at all.

When an attack does strike, the pain is more prolonged than with angina, because the arterial blockage is greater.

How is the possibility of a heart attack established?

Principally through electrocardiograms (ECGs), although doctors also take into consideration such factors as age, weight, blood pressure, and cholesterol level.

Supplementing the ECGs are such diagnostic tools as blood tests, angiograms, and radionuclide imaging.

If a heart attack does strike, what are the chances of survival, and how is the condition treated?

Although heart disease is America's number one killer, the good news is that 90 percent of the people who make it through the first few days after an attack can expect a full recovery. The key to survival is being quickly admitted to a hospital's cardiac-care unit. Perhaps the first medication you'll receive there will be aspirin, to help dissolve the blood clots causing the problem, followed by drugs ranging from morphine to beta-blockers to other anticoagulants. Oxygen may also be administered.

It's possible that the cardiac specialists will decide, within the first few hours, that your condition can be handled exclusively through medication. Thrombolytic therapy, for instance, calls for heavy doses of such anticoagulants as streptokinase and urokinase.

Alternatively, the doctors may feel you'll be better served by an angioplasty or even by a coronary bypass, in which veins or arteries from elsewhere in your body are grafted onto the blocked artery, "bypassing" the obstruction.

What kind of rehabilitation comes next?

Cardiac-care specialists will try to get you on your feet within a couple of days, and out of the hospital within a week. Then, under close supervision, you'll be put on a graduated exercise program for the next couple of months to forestall further clotting. Simultaneously, your doctor will be urging you to think long-term and preaching the benefits of a low-fat diet, no tobacco, and continued exercise.

What complications can a heart-attack patient expect?

They're myriad, ranging from habitual weak heartbeats that require strong medication to out-of-sync heartbeats that require pacemaker implants. Luckily, most of the complications have solutions.

How do blood clots occur?

The blood in your arteries and veins thickens, or clots, if the blood vessel is opened or otherwise damaged, and that's normal. But clots, also known as embolisms, that form within the arteries and veins because of disease or impaired circulation (and then break away to lodge themselves elsewhere within the circulatory system) are abnormal, often causing severe pain, dizziness, and nausea. Clots in the coronary arteries can bring on heart attacks. Clots in the cerebral artery can bring on a stroke.

How are they treated?

With aspirin and anticoagulants, sometimes surgery, and then the usual regimen of high-fiber, low-fat diet, no smoking, and plenty of exercise.

Can you sum up the kinds of medications that are prescribed for patients who have had heart attacks or are in danger of having them?

There are several categories of drugs, all of which have to be carefully monitored to prevent injurious side effects:

- Diuretics—water pills—reduce high blood pressure and at the same time relieve the symptoms of congestive heart failure, which occurs when the heart's pumping action is so weak that fluid backs up into the lungs.

- ACE inhibitors, which block the hormones that constrict blood vessels, are effective in relieving hypertension.

- Calcium channel blockers keep calcium from being released into the muscles, thereby relaxing the blood vessels and lowering blood pressure.

- Beta-blockers, which reduce the heart rate and the amount of oxygen the heart uses, lessen the likelihood of a second heart attack and ease the pain caused by angina.

- Cholesterol-lowering drugs, especially the so-called statin medications, are particularly effective in preventing heart attacks.

- Aspirin, which keeps the blood cells from clotting, staves off heart disease and strokes.

Are clot-busting drugs safe for older people?

Clot-busting drugs are quite effective in emergency treatment of heart attacks. If they are taken within twelve hours after an attack, they can even dissolve the blockages in coronary arteries that have been narrowed by arteriosclerosis. Until recently they were thought to help older patients just as much as younger ones. Now some studies have found that the drugs may fail to help people age seventy-five and older and may indeed put them at higher risk.

Some one million Americans suffer heart attacks annually, and about one-third of them are over seventy-five years of age.

Both the American Heart Association and the American College of Cardiology warn that the effectiveness and the safety of clot busters for such patients are debatable. The two main prescription drugs in this category are tPA (tissue plasminogen activator) and streptokinase.

One of the studies, from Johns Hopkins, involved some 8,000 patients ages sixty-five to eighty-six. Statistics showed that 18 percent of heart-attack victims ages seventy-six to eighty-six who received clot busters died within thirty days of treatment, compared with 15.4 percent of those not given the drugs. Among patients ages sixty-five to seventy-five, however, the negative numbers became positive. Those who received clot busters had a thirty-day death rate of 6.8 percent, compared with 9.8 percent of patients who were not given the medications.

I've heard that giving heart-attack victims chest compression alone is as effective as combining it with mouth-to-mouth resuscitation. Is this true?

Researchers at the University of Washington recently found that simple compression is just as effective as full-blown CPR. This study, which involved some 240 people receiving emergency aid, found no statistical difference in survival rates between the two groups. Pumping the blood through the arteries solely by chest compression, the researchers stated, usually circulated sufficient oxygen to keep the brain alive until an ambulance arrived.

The study also concluded that simple compression might be the more efficient of the two techniques, given that full CPR requires too much time to explain over the phone in an emergency.

Can angioplasties be delayed safely?

For the best survival rate, angioplasties should be performed within two hours after the patient arrives at the hospital. If treatment is delayed any longer, death rates can rise by 40 to 60 percent.

Moreover, patients who receive emergency angioplasties at hospitals that perform a large number of such procedures likewise have better survival rates—their chances improve as much as 25 to 30 percent.

What effect does exercise have on the blood vessels?

Exercise is generally beneficial to the body, of course, but now we also know that it specifically strengthens the blood vessels—particularly among older people. This is because the efficacy of the mechanism releasing nitrous oxide into the bloodstream is to a greater or lesser degree impaired as we age, particularly if we are sedentary. Nitrous oxide protects the vessels against clogging and dilutes them when the heart requires more blood.

Researchers recently looked at two groups of people pursuing vigorous exercise programs, one whose average age was twenty-seven and one whose average age was sixty-three. Their conclusion: Largely because of exercise, nitrous oxide was released into the vessels of the older group just as efficiently as in the younger group.

Chronic Fatigue Syndrome (CFS)

Is this syndrome fact or fancy?

Definitely fact. Besides being chronically tired, patients endure an array of flulike symptoms for months, even several years, on end. Neither rest nor medication brings about a cure. Then, as suddenly as it strikes, the disease plays itself out.

Who does CFS hit?

Mostly professional people under forty, and twice as many women as men.

What are the causes?

Nobody knows, though it's not for lack of theorizing—usually about the immune system. The Epstein-Barr virus, which brings on mononucleosis, was once the prime suspect but has since been exonerated. Hypotheses now range from more mysterious herpes viruses to mundane fungal infections in the mouth or vagina, from overuse of antibiotics to overexposure to pesticides.

How is CFS treated?

We treat the flulike symptoms and the fatigue separately, then watch and wait.

Aspirin may relieve the headache and fever, anti-inflammatories the muscle soreness, and monoamine oxidase inhibitors the tendency toward insomnia.

To mitigate the fatigue factor and bolster the immune system, we advise getting plenty of rest, eating sensibly and drinking alcohol sparingly, avoiding stressful situations, and relaxing the muscles with gentle exercise.

What about vitamins and food supplements?

Vitamin A (beta-carotene), vitamin B_6, manganese, and zinc may be effective in relieving fatigue, while garlic tablets may stimulate the immune system.

Conjunctivitis

The conjunctiva is a thin lining that protects the white of the eye and covers the back of the eyelid. If it becomes inflamed, the result is pain, redness, and itching.

Are there different types of conjunctivitis?

Conjunctivitis can be caused by bacterial or viral agents or by allergic reactions.

If it's bacterial, usually both eyes are affected and the discharge is thick and creamy; if it's viral, only one eye tears up, and the discharge is clear; if the conjunctivitis is allergic, both eyes tear up, the discharge is clear, and the nose also runs.

How long does the disease last?

Conjunctivitis generally is not serious but can last for months, first receding, then flaring up again. If bacterial or viral, the disease is, however, highly contagious. Wash your hands before and after bathing or treating the eye, and do not share hand towels.

What is the usual treatment?

Usually antibiotic drops or ointment for bacterial conjunctivitis, antihistamine tablets or corticosteroid drops for viral and allergic conditions.

Caution: Corticosteroids should not be taken if a herpes infection is suspected.

Constipation and Diarrhea

How often should I have a bowel movement?

It varies with the individual: One person may require more than one movement a day, another may be comfortable with only one movement every couple of days.

Understand, however, that the longer the fecal matter stays in the intestine, the harder it becomes. If you chronically have difficulty passing your stools, you should change your dietary habits.

What do you mean?

- Put more fiber in your diet—fruits, vegetables, and cereals—to help soften your stools.

- Make sure you exercise daily, to keep loose and relaxed.

How do I cope with the opposite problem—diarrhea?

As with constipation, everyone occasionally suffers from diarrhea. It's only when the symptoms become chronic—heavy, watery movements over time—that you should restrict your food intake.

Sometimes the problem may be too much coffee or too many cola drinks in your diet, too much sugar, or even too much fiber.

Can chronic constipation and diarrhea indicate some more serious disease?

They may portend serious abdominal problems. See your doctor.

Cornea Injuries

The cornea is the convex portion of the outer eyeball, filled with cells and fluid, that protects the iris and pupil.

What does it mean to "scratch" one's eye?

This often refers to an abrasion of the cornea. Because the eye is so rich in nerve endings, the pain is exquisite and is heightened by the loss of eye fluid and excessive blinking.

How do I lessen the discomfort?

To avoid further abrasion of the cornea, avoid rubbing your eye. Use hydrating drops to reduce the painful effects of drying and, if necessary, an eye patch to retard blinking and promote healing.

If the pain persists or your vision is impaired, you may require an antibiotic and a painkiller.

Dependency

What is dependency?

Dependency is an overreliance on something or someone and is a self-destructive behavior pattern.

Patients who become too dependent on drugs, for instance, impair their mental clarity, personal relationships, job performance, and, ultimately, their health. Patients who become too dependent on others—whether overreliant on doctors, therapists, or spouses—undermine their own ability to control their lives.

Everyone needs help, but leaning too heavily on external supports, instead of oneself, is most unwise.

But surely it's not wrong to depend on family and friends in times of crisis?

Of course not. Two-way relationships, based on mutual love and interaction, can be a great comfort to sufferers. But one-way relationships, those in which people expect help unilaterally, taking but not giving, are another matter. Ultimately, they end in anger, accusations, even abandonment.

I'm constantly worrying, "What if the pain gets worse? . . . What if I can't work? . . . What if my family stops loving me?" Does this mean I'm lapsing into dependency?

Not at all. The "what if" cycle, played and replayed in the sufferer's mind, is completely normal, though it must be resisted. Obsessive thoughts lead to erroneous conclusions. Resolve to lay aside your worries, first for one hour, then two, then a longer period. Recite, over and over, the Tibetan proverb "Just for today I will not worry."

What is codependency?

Codependency is the personification of the one-way relationship and has detrimental consequences for both parties.

The initial lure is that one person is helping and the other is being helped. By creating codependency, however, neither party functions in a self-directed fashion. The relationship is, therefore, ultimately doomed.

How can the cycle of dependency be broken?

Self-reliance can be achieved through education, creative activities, meditation, support groups, accumulated life experiences, and similar positive steps.

Depression

Depression is the most common psychological problem in the United States, affecting some 18 million people annually. But clinical depression isn't merely "feeling low." It's a real disease, with persistent symptoms; and even after the disease is treated, it has a high recurrence rate.

What are the symptoms?

Depression sufferers can experience headaches, chest pains, stomach and abdominal pains, muscle aches, and, yes, just about any symptom you can name. The mind is capable of creating the perception of pain in any part of the body.

Moreover, if these psychological pain symptoms are unchecked, real physical deterioration can occur. The mind and body are intensely linked.

But is the pain in my mind or in my body?

Does it matter? It's like arguing about which came first, the chicken or the egg.

The depressed mind produces a negative outlook that changes reality, drains the body's resources, creates physical illness. Sufferers experience both emotional and bodily pain. The former must be clinically explored; the latter, treated and, if possible, reversed.

We accept patients' perception of their pain and try to shape and reduce the discomfort by helping them understand its cause. Rejecting the patients' perception would only increase their isolation.

Are there different types of depression?

Reactive depressions are minor, caused by external events. They occur when we lose a loved one or learn that we have a debilitating illness. They mostly run a defined, temporary course: the initial shock, a period of depression, then the healing.

Endogenous depressions are major, coming from within. Innate psychic pressures overwhelm us, bringing insomnia, listlessness, feelings of worthlessness. They seem unending. Day after day, we remain shrouded in gloom.

What therapies ease the pain of endogenous, or major, depression?

Treatment usually consists of a combination of antidepressant drugs and professional counseling.

The antidepressants, which seek to change the neurochemical imbalances that cause our gloom, fall into three categories: serotonin inhibitors, which affect the neurochemical of the same name; tricyclics; and monoamine oxidase inhibitors.

Counseling depends on how deep-rooted the disease is, ranging from rigorous probing by a psychiatrist to less invasive advice from a psychotherapist.

Can you tell me more about these medications?

Low levels of the neurotransmitter serotonin are thought to be linked to depressed moods. Selective serotonin reuptake inhibitors (SSRIs) like Prozac increase the level of the chemical in the brain, hopefully elevating the patient's spirits and usually producing few side effects.

Tricyclics like Tofranil, so-called because their molecules are composed of three rings, are often described as tried-and-true anti-depressants. But their side effects can be considerable. Drawbacks may include drowsiness, impaired vision, constipation, difficulty in urinating, and dizziness.

Monoamine oxidase (MAO) inhibitors like Nardil likewise attempt to elevate moods by blocking the action of a chemical in the brain. One side effect of this type of medication is that the liver can no longer metabolize tyramine. This means that tyramine-rich foods like cheese and herring must be avoided.

How do I know whether the medication my doctor prescribes is strong enough?

Be patient. You should let four to six weeks pass before asking for a stronger dosage. The more powerful the dosage, the greater the chance of unpleasant side effects.

Moreover, once you start taking a particular antidepressant, you should realize that you are making a commitment. It may be nine to twelve months before the drug finally takes effect.

It's important you keep your physician informed of your progress. Then you can jointly decide on the dosage and medication that's best for your individual case.

What alternative therapies do you recommend?

Our favorite is exercise. Whether you walk, jog, run, swim, or play tennis or golf is immaterial. Just do something every day. Exercise stimulates blood flow to the brain, temporarily relieving your problem.

Other alternative treatments include religious or philosophical meditation, self-guided imagery, and music or art therapy.

A cautionary note: Bear in mind that alcohol intake greatly aggravates depression, as do tranquilizers like Valium.

How does my depression affect those around me?

Depressed people often project a negative aura, so it's not surprising that they get negative feedback. Abrupt, rude, or agitated behavior invites like responses. The result is an impasse, at both home and work, in which everyone loses.

We urge patients to turn negative actions, however slowly, into positive ones. Your depression may be too deep to attack the problem head-on, but with professional help, you should be able to initiate small changes, then work up to more substantial ones.

I feel "blue" about half the time. Am I in danger of falling into major depression?

You may be, particularly if you don't know why you're feeling depressed. Some days are diamonds, some days are stones, but if you find yourself "blue" on occasions others find enjoyable, you may need counseling.

Dermatitis

This inflammation causes skin itching, dryness, and redness. Symptoms may be aggravated by hot compresses, relieved by cold ones.

What types of dermatitis are there?

There are numerous subdivisions. Contact dermatitis is a reaction to a specific substance—the chemicals in cosmetics, the nickel in jewelry, the chemicals used in making clothing and shoes. Finding and removing the irritant is the first step in treatment, then using hydrocortisone cream for mild cases.

Nummular dermatitis, which hits older people, usually consists of round, red patches on the extremities. It responds well to salt water and corticosteroid creams. Seborrheic dermatitis is found in the scalp area. Coal tar–based shampoos are beneficial.

I have a great deal of scaling around my ankles. Is this a form of dermatitis?

You may have stasis dermatitis, which tends to affect people with varicose veins. The blood is partially blocked from returning up the veins and pools around the ankles, causing scaling and irritation. Elevating your legs is helpful.

My rashes tend to blister, then show signs of infection. Is this dermatitis?

You may have atopic dermatitis, or eczema. Besides the appropriate creams, treatment may call for antibiotics.

What is scleroderma?

It's an autoimmune disorder that until recently was considered untreatable; it affects some 75,000 to 100,000 Americans, mostly women of childbearing age. Fibrous tissue like collagen grows unchecked, leaving the skin tight and shiny and eventually causing abnormalities in the organs and blood vessels.

Now researchers at the University of Medicine and Dentistry of New Jersey and the Robert Wood Johnson Medical School in New Brunswick have hopes of treating the disease with a form of the hormone relaxin, which is produced during pregnancy and prevents the growth of fibrous tissue. Patients who received relaxin began showing improvement within four weeks of treatment, and half of them had their skin symptoms reduced by a third.

Diabetes and Hypoglycemia

Diabetes mellitus is caused by the body's insufficiently producing insulin, the hormone that converts blood sugar (or glucose) into energy, resulting in elevated blood-sugar levels.

Are there different kinds of diabetes mellitus?

There are two variations. In Type I diabetes, which mostly affects people under thirty, little or no insulin is produced. In Type II diabetes, which generally affects people over forty, the body does not process insulin properly.

The Type II condition is by far the most common, accounting for nine out of every ten sufferers, of whom perhaps 90 percent are substantially overweight.

What are the symptoms?

Thirst, frequent urination, hunger, drowsiness, and blurred vision are among the warning signs.

How is a diagnosis made?

Usually through a blood test, taken early in the morning before the patient has had anything to eat or drink.

And the treatment?

Understand that the way to handle diabetes is to keep blood-sugar levels within normal parameters (or as close to them as possible).

The way we do this, for Type I diabetics who lack sufficient insulin, is through self-administered insulin injections. (Because stomach juices nullify insulin's effects, it can't be taken orally.) Tiny syringes with thin needles make the procedure all but painless.

Type II diabetics, who produce insulin but process it badly, may or may not need injections.

In both instances, however, patients must follow a regimen involving regular eating habits and exercise.

How often are the injections needed?

That depends on the individual and on how closely the condition needs to be monitored. Rapid-acting insulin takes effect in thirty minutes but lasts only six hours; intermediate, in two to four hours but lasts twenty-four hours; long-acting, in six hours but lasts thirty-six hours.

The closest control is attained by injecting a rapid as well as an intermediate dosage each morning, then taking rapid-acting dosages the rest of the day.

What kind of eating and exercise are advisable?

Generally speaking, you should restrict your intake of sugars and fats, eat small but regular meals, and, if you're overweight, take off the poundage as soon as possible.

Type I diabetics, to keep blood-sugar levels normal, should consume three small meals and three snacks daily, with carbohydrates constituting half of their diet. Having a snack before moderate exercise is particularly important. Type II diabetics should pursue a similar program.

Studies have shown that a high-carbohydrate, high-fiber diet can reduce the need for insulin by anywhere from 30 to 100 percent.

Can fiber intake help arrest the onset of diabetes?

Many experts think so. Researchers at the University of Texas Southwestern Medical Center and the Veterans Affairs Medical Center, both in Dallas, recently put diabetic patients on a six-week high-fiber diet. During this period the patients' daily glucose concentrations dropped by 10 percent, and other measurements of the disease were similarly reduced.

Is the incidence of diabetes rising?

In the past decade there has been a 76 percent increase in Type II diabetes among people in their thirties, and many researchers warn that the disease will take a drastic toll in the years to come. They attribute the problem to inactivity in front of TV screens and computer sets, lack of consistent exercise, and overeating—particularly of fatty and junk foods.

In the past, Type II diabetes was found primarily in people over forty-five. Now obese individuals in their thirties, and even teenagers, are targets of the disease. Not every obese person becomes a diabetic, of course, but the risk is in direct proportion to the degree of excess poundage. Researchers speculate that obesity increases the level of blood sugar, or glucose, and brings about insulin resistance. If the body does not make proper use of insulin, the hormone that helps glucose fuel the cells, diabetes results.

Can too much insulin lower the blood-sugar level too much?

Yes, an overdose of insulin can cause severe complications, as can not eating on time or not snacking before exercising. The condition is called hypoglycemia, which is marked by sweating, shaking, and faintness.

How can hypoglycemia be treated?

By promptly ingesting some sugar, whether candy, fruit juice, or sugared water.

What other complications does diabetes threaten?

Unless tightly monitored, diabetes increases the chance of heart disease, weakens eyesight, impairs the kidneys, and causes skin infections.

What is a common pain syndrome that diabetics experience?

Diabetic neuropathic pain and peripheral neuropathy are nerve dysfunctions causing a sensory pain signal. Some oral agents are available to treat such pain. Physicians disagree about whether diabetic management can alleviate this type of nerve dysfunction.

Ear Pain

Earaches occur when there is inflammation in either the outer or middle ear, or when there is undue pressure on the eardrum, which separates the two channels.

Why is ear pain so debilitating?

The sensory organs are particularly rich in nerve endings, so the pain is heightened. It may spread to the face and, sometimes, the throat. Nausea and even vertigo may result.

What are the usual therapies?

To deal with excess earwax putting pressure on the eardrum, try warm washes of hydrogen peroxide several times daily.

To reduce inflammation, antibiotic ear drops may be prescribed, as may steroids.

Acetaminophen (Tylenol) will ease the pain.

I do a lot of air travel, and I always have an earache when we're landing. What can I do about it?

The sudden change in air pressure is causing the eardrum to bulge inward. Close your nostrils and gently blow air to correct the imbalance.

Why do children get so many ear infections?

Ear infections, or otitis media, stem from the eustachian tube being blocked, usually as a result of the colds or respiratory ailments so common among children. Fluid accumulates in the middle ear, forming a breeding ground for bacteria.

One recent study in the *British Medical Journal* suggests that otitis media can be greatly reduced by giving children two sticks of gum made with the sweetener xylitol after every meal or snack. Children taking xylitol in this manner had 40 percent fewer ear infections than those who did not.

Xylitol is a natural substance derived from birch trees and is thought to block the growth of *Streptococcus pneumoniae,* the most common cause of otitis media.

Epilepsy

What is epilepsy?

It's a neurological disorder in the brain, an irritation if you will, that creates abnormal electrical activity and causes recurring seizures.

What brings on the condition?

Sometimes the culprit is a brain injury at birth, an inherited gene, drugs, or even harsh lighting. Sometimes we just don't know.

How is the disorder diagnosed?

Generally through the use of an electroencephalogram (EEG), a pain-less procedure. We attach electrodes around the scalp, then monitor the brain's wave patterns under both normal and abnormal circumstances.

Are there different kinds of epilepsy?

The attacks can be either general, affecting the whole brain, or partial, affecting a specific area. Most seizures are general and are further subdivided into either petit mal or grand mal conditions.

Petit mal attacks usually begin in childhood and are characterized by vacant staring, repetitious swallowing, and facial twitching. Grand mal attacks involve loss of consciousness, violent spasms, and tongue biting.

Perhaps the best-known partial seizures are temporal lobe and jacksonian attacks. The former, occurring in the area of the brain associated with the sense of smell, bring on various mental aberrations. The latter involve muscle twitching in the arms or legs.

How is the disease treated?

Usually through anticonvulsant drugs, such as phenobarbital, phenytoin, and primidone. Such medications can be highly effective, preventing or drastically reducing the frequency of (e.g., by two-thirds) grand mal attacks.

Are the anticonvulsant drugs taken in combination?

As a rule of thumb, it's best to treat epilepsy with a single medication. This doesn't mean, of course, that you're tied to one drug in perpetuity. But you should give one medication time to alleviate your symptoms before switching to another. Otherwise, you're simply sending the brain mixed signals. For some people, combination therapy is clearly indicated.

Is surgery ever called for?

Only if drugs are useless, the seizures are constant, and the irritated part of the brain is clearly identified and closely confined.

What pain syndromes to seizure sufferers experience?

A very common pain syndrome that epileptics experience is gingivitis (gum hyperplasia), the gum dysfunction associated with intake of anticonvulsant medication. The best setting to evaluate the use of such medication is with the treating physician/neurologist.

Flu

Influenza, the virus spread by touching infected people or inhaling infected droplets in the air, is the mother of all colds. Sneezing, coughing, aches, and fever debilitate the patient.

How do I make it through the flu season?

The best way to deal with the flu is prevention: flu shots may be a necessity, especially if your job calls for you to interact with a large number of people.

But what if I get the flu?

You'll have to let it run its course, which is usually a week or two. Because the flu is viral in origin, antibiotics are no help.

Try over-the-counter cough medicines, some with codeine additives, and analgesics. Get as much rest as possible and avoid dehydration by drinking lots of liquids.

Why do I feel so weak?

The virus creates a systemic infection throughout the body. Fever and coughing further weaken the patient and may lead to physical exhaustion.

Gingivitis and Periodontitis

This disease, whose symptoms are red and swollen gums, is the result of poor dental hygiene.

What can I do about it?

You should brush and floss regularly, perhaps several times a day. This prevents the buildup of bacteria-laden plaque, which, if left on the gums, will harden into tartar, requiring professional removal.

Frequent warm salt-water rinses will ease the pain.

Can gingivitis lead to tooth loss?

Yes, if it evolves into periodontitis, in which the plaque and tartar buildup is big enough to pull the tooth away from the gum and, eventually, from the bone. Periodontal problems require clinical attention.

Are there any new developments in treating gum disease that will help me avoid the pain and expense of periodontia?

Gum disease is caused by bacteria invading the area between the tooth and gum. Unless you get treatment, bone erosion and tooth loss will result.

Now a group of antibiotic drugs may be on the point of replacing, or at least making more effective, the painful scaling and root planing, which often requires local anesthesia. These drugs either are taken orally or are placed in the diseased pocket between the tooth and gum. Ronada Davis, a dentist at Texas Medical Center in Houston, recommends Atridox, an antibiotic gel. Though she has treated some 200 patients with "great success," she acknowledges that she has "run into few periodontists who use it. Obviously they want to do surgery."

Atridox was approved by the Food and Drug Administration in 1998. It is injected between the gum and tooth, where it hardens and then gradually releases the antibiotic doxycycline over a two-week period.

Atridox is thus far the only drug recommended for stand-alone treatment; other currently available antibiotics are used only after scaling and root planing. One of these, Periostat, is a pill containing a low dose of doxycycline. The dose is not strong enough to kill bacteria, but it does suppress the enzymes that destroy collagen. A recent study in the *Journal of Periodontology* reported that taken after scaling and planing, Periostat reduced the disease pockets far more efficaciously than surgery alone. In some cases the progression of gum disease was 90 percent lower.

When will this type of antibiotic treatment be generally available to periodontitis sufferers?

Many doctors and dentists feel that their everyday use is long overdue. Rick Niederman, head of the Office of Evidence-Based Dentistry at the Harvard School of Dental Medicine, is currently collaborating with Delta Dental Plan of Massachusetts on a study comparing surgical and nonsurgical techniques. Dr. Niederman says the dental profession is moving toward antibiotics, but slowly. "We are in a transition period," he explains.

Do you know of any other improvements in the treatment of gum disease?

The same University of California at San Francisco biotechnology group that is transforming human skin into bone and cartilage (see "Arthritis") has transformed a type of gum cell—the gingival fibroblast—into jawbone. Recently CeraMed Dental, a small company owned by Dentsply International, secured Food and Drug Administration approval to sell a product based on the research. CeraMed's product is called PepGen P-15. In FDA trials PepGen P-15 generated new growth in the jaw in roughly three-quarters of the areas where it was used.

Gout

What is gout?

It's a form of arthritis. Crystals formed by abnormally high levels of uric acid in the blood accumulate in the joints, notably the toes and ankles, inflaming them and bringing on intense pain and swelling.

Whom does the disease strike?

The overwhelming number of sufferers are middle-aged men, about half of whom have a genetic propensity toward the problem.

What triggers the attacks?

They often result from overindulgence in fatty foods and alcohol, which raises the level of uric acid to the point where it can't be passed from the body in the urine.

What therapies exist?

Colchicine is a long-standing medication used to reduce the inflammation, but it can have adverse side effects, particularly if you are simultaneously taking antidepressants, antihistamines, or tranquilizers.

Today your doctor is more likely to prescribe nonsteroidal anti-inflammatory drugs (NSAIDs) such as ibuprofen, or even corticosteroids such as prednisone.

Do dietary changes help?

Rich, fatty foods should be avoided, of course, as should those high in protein. Drink plenty of nonalcoholic liquids, at least several quarts daily.

If you are obese, start losing weight.

What can I do immediately to ease the pain?

Gently place a bag of ice cubes over the joint. This should temporarily reduce the inflammation.

Are there alternative therapies?

Both acupressure and acupuncture can be beneficial. Acupressure has the advantage, once a professional shows you the proper pressure points, of being able to be self-administered at home.

Grief

Is grieving a good thing?

Grieving is a healthy component of dealing with death, separation, loss, and severe illness. When grief is cut short, one cannot adapt appropriately.

However, when grief is prolonged, a destructive cycle can evolve, bringing on hopelessness, deep depression, and social isolation.

How can I help a loved one trapped in prolonged grief?

It's difficult. Your loved one's grief is so entrenched that you cannot attack it directly. That tactic will only result in anger and resentment.

Try to help the loved one see, in a series of small steps, the self-destructive nature of the grief. Accept that the healing process will be progressive and slow.

What are some ways to break the cycle of grieving?

Diversions such as films, concerts, and plays have significant healing qualities. So do physical activities ranging from yoga to aerobics, from dancing to tennis. They take the grief-stricken out of themselves, curtailing negative thoughts.

Support groups are invaluable, helping people to ventilate and recognize that others have gone through similar experiences.

Hand Injuries

Why did it take so long to recover when I injured my hand?

The hand is made up of a complex network of tendons, nerves, muscles, and blood vessels, all in a densely packed and unforgiving space. It grasps, grabs, and pinches; curves and twists the fingers; and manipulates objects. Its movements require strength, skill, and motor control. Even slight damage to the hand upsets its coordination.

Why is edema in the hand so dangerous?

Accumulated fluids readily disrupt the knuckle and pulling mechanisms of the hand. If the fluids turn toxic, they can cause permanent damage.

Is it more serious to injure my right, or more dominant, hand than my left hand?

It's pretty much a toss-up. While most of us rely on our right hands to write, cut our meat, or comb our hair, our left hands simultaneously act as a guide—to position the notebook, hold the fork, or pat down the hair. Damage to either hand makes the small tasks more difficult and the big ones impossible.

Why does the arthritis in my hands bother me so?

The arthritis serves as a painful, constant reminder of how dependent you are on your hands.

Repetition may be the aggravating factor in your condition. The repetitive tasks you perform daily, at work and at home, may be irritating your joints and tendons and, in effect, fueling your arthritis.

Today there are all manner of devices specifically designed to relieve this stress. They range from user-friendly keyboards to easily grasped handles to more efficient tools and utensils. Ask your doctor about them.

What other therapies exist for arthritic hand pain?

Splinting individual fingers or the entire hand can be beneficial. This treatment, by itself, may not cure the condition, but it eases the pain. At the same time, it's far better than simply relying on painkillers, and risking dependency.

Other therapies range from anti-inflammatory drugs to soaking your hands in warm water.

When is surgery necessary?

Severe damage to the tendons and bones may require surgical transplants, attachments, or alignments. The ensuing physical therapy calls for "reeducating" the hand, step-by-step, so it can regain its many functions.

Hay Fever

Prolonged sneezing, itchy roof of the mouth, watery eyes, runny nose—these are all the symptoms of hay fever. The ailment, a response to various airborne pollens, technically is called allergic rhinitis.

Why do I get hay fever in the spring, and my friend gets it in the autumn?

Most hay fever victims suffer from seasonal allergies. If your symptoms occur in the spring, you're sensitive to pollen from trees; in the summer, from grasses; in the autumn, from ragweed; in the winter, from fungus spores.

Some people, we regret to say, suffer from perennial allergies, spanning all or most of the year.

Why does the body react so violently to the airborne pollens?

Your immune system, for reasons we do not fully understand, overreacts. It sees the pollens as menacing intruders and produces a counteragent called histamine, which irritates the sinuses and brings on your miseries.

What are the usual medications?

There is a wide range of effective antihistamines: some prescription, like dexchlorpheniramine and trimeprazine; some over-the-counter, like chlorpheniramine and phenindamine. Decongestants, like pseudoephedrine, are also useful.

Nasal sprays, many containing cromolyn sodium, relieve itchiness in the nose and on the roof of the mouth. In severe cases, sprays containing corticosteroids are suggested.

What are some of the commonly used prescription antihistamines?

Claritin and Allegra are currently two of the most effective oral medications. They need to be taken only once a day, and most people experience relief within the hour.

Flonase is an excellent nasal spray. Once the allergic symptoms are relieved, it too need be administered only once daily.

How effective is immunotherapy?

Immunotherapy involves injecting the allergy substance under the skin, in larger and larger doses, until the body no longer reacts to it. While this procedure can be beneficial, it may not be cost-effective, provided the allergy can be treated more simply.

Headache—Migraine

Migraines strike less than 15 percent of the population but result in some 157 million lost workdays annually, again according to the National Headache Foundation.

How do migraines differ from tension headaches?

Migraines are usually vascular in origin, with the alternate constricting and swelling of the blood vessels producing a throbbing pain. Sufferers, who are extremely sensitive to light, noise, and odors, experience severe discomfort around their eyes and nose.

Attacks, which can be quite debilitating, may occur each time in a regular pattern, with the onsets being signaled by "light flashes" or nausea.

Is a migraine always a migraine?

Many people attach the label *migraine* to all headaches. Understand that migraine symptoms require professional evaluation and testing, usually by a neurologist. Patients commonly receive MRIs or CAT scans of their head before any diagnosis is made.

What are some remedies for migraines?

As with tension headaches, simple treatments include applying cool compresses and avoiding intense light and noise.

Infrequent migraines may call for such drugs as ergotamine, which narrows the blood vessels, or sumatriptan, which has a similar effect. Frequent migraines (three or more a month) call for preventive medications, such as propranolol or verapamil, that likewise affect the vascular system but can be taken on a regular basis.

Which of these drugs have the fewest side effects?

Probably sumatriptan, which is sold under the name Imitrex. It can be taken orally or injected, and though it is designed to cope with moderate migraines, it can also be effective against more frequent attacks. Imitrex produces few of the side effects of comparable drugs—nausea, sleepiness, and dependence—but you should expect some flushing.

For best results, the medication should be taken as soon as possible after the migraine strikes.

Do migraine sufferers get their headaches at predictable times, perhaps the same day of the week?

Interesting that you should ask. A study conducted by the Palm Beach Medical Center in Florida recently found that migraines struck teenagers most often on Mondays and only rarely on Saturdays. But the researchers insisted that the statistics were not evidence of malingering.

"We suspect the finding may have to do with the anxiety of getting ready to go to school, or perhaps changing sleep patterns," said Dr. Paul Winner, codirector of the center.

Can the eye pain in migraines signal some other disorder?

Yes. Eye pain can also be a symptom of more serious ophthalmic or central-nervous-system diseases. Particularly when it's persistent or recurrent, such discomfort requires prompt medical attention.

Headache—Tension

If you feel as if someone is tightening a clamp around your head, and the pain is steady and nonthrobbing, you have a tension headache. But you're in good, if unhappy, company. Some 65 to 70 percent of the population endures tension headaches, according to the National Headache Foundation.

Is this problem always caused by "tension"?

Stress can be a major cause. But this type of headache is also precipitated by unsound diet, toxins, sleep disturbances, noise, bad lighting, and a host of other factors.

What causes the tightness in my brow and the back of my neck?

We are all familiar with the muscles in our torso and limbs. But there are also muscles beneath the skin of the face and neck, giving us the ability to create facial expressions and turn our heads. Contraction in these muscles causes our pain.

What simple remedies are available for tension headaches?

Cool compresses, low lighting, gentle finger pressure over the tight and painful areas.

What steps can I take at home and at work to lessen my discomfort?

Try to live and work in a moderately lit, minimally noisy environment. Try to avoid such pain triggers as TV and computer glare, traffic and factory din, any sight or sound too intense or too harsh.

What medications ease tension headaches, and what substances exacerbate them?

Aspirin and analgesics like acetaminophen are common remedies. Acetaminophen-only drugs include such brand names as Tylenol; acetaminophen in combination with other drugs includes Chlor-Trimeton, Contac, DayQuil, and NyQuil. To avoid withdrawal pangs, use the least potent, not the most potent, remedy you can.

Excessive caffeine and sugar, as well as alcohol and nicotine, should be shunned. But a glass of warm milk will do wonders for the problem.

What if my headaches persist?

Tension headaches should be transient. If they persist, your doctor should perform further tests.

Hemorrhoids

Hemorrhoidal veins, located both within and at the base of the rectum, can easily become swollen, resulting in pain, itching, and sometimes bleeding.

What causes hemorrhoids?

Some people may inherit weak veins in the anal area, just as others inherit weak, or varicose, veins in their legs.

Essentially, however, the problem is one of poor diet. People who eschew fruits and vegetables, which are high-fiber foods, often develop constipation. The ensuing strain during bowel movements, and the passing of hard stools, irritate and swell the veins.

What temporary remedies exist?

Sitting in the bathtub, in several inches of warm water several times a day, will shrink the veins and ease the discomfort. Over-the-counter anesthetic ointments may also be beneficial.

But changing one's dietary habits, and drinking adequate amounts of fluid, is the basic solution.

Do hemorrhoids sometimes require surgery?

Large internal hemorrhoids may, particularly if the blood is clotting and the pain is especially severe.

Hepatitis

What is hepatitis?
It's a viral inflammation of the liver. Symptoms include fever, fatigue, and loss of appetite.

How is it commonly transmitted?
Hepatitis A is usually caused by poor hygeine—not washing one's hands after a bowel movement, for example, and then preparing food—as is hepatitis E, which triggers epidemics in Third World countries.

Hepatitis B (and its more severe cousin, hepatitis D) occurs among drug users who share needles and among promiscuous sexual partners who do not use contraceptives.

The chief cause of hepatitis C is contaminated blood transfusions.

Nonviral forms of hepatitis, it should be noted, can spring from drug and alcohol abuse.

How is the disease diagnosed?
Through blood tests and, sometimes, by performing a biopsy—taking a tiny bit of tissue from the liver and having it analyzed.

What therapies exist?
Basically the disease has to run its course. Get as much rest as you can, eat a nutritious diet, and avoid alcohol. The acute stage usually lasts a couple of weeks; complete recovery takes a couple of months.

Chronic cases of hepatitis B and C may be treated with interferon, which strengthens the body's resistance to infection and lessens the chance of cirrhosis, or serious liver damage.

What foods are best?

Fibrous foods, including cereals, fruits, leafy vegetables, and a wide variety of beans. They clean out the toxins that are irritating the liver.

What are the best preventive measures?

- Be hygiene-conscious at all times.

- Be careful about making intimate contact with people whose blood or bodily fluids you suspect may be contaminated.

Hiatal Hernia

Is it true that most people with a hiatal hernia don't realize they have one?

That's correct. Symptoms include aching in the chest, regurgitation, and a bloated feeling; most sufferers confuse the problem with heartburn.

Precisely what is a hiatal hernia?

The esophagus, the tube that brings food down from the mouth and throat, enters the stomach through the hiatus, a small opening in the diaphragm, the muscle separating the stomach from the chest.

Hiatal hernias occur when the lower esophagus and part of the stomach push upward through the hiatus and diaphragm, ballooning in various configurations into the chest cavity.

Are there different kinds?

The two most common are sliding hiatal hernia, in which part of the stomach pushes through the hiatus into the esophagus proper, and paraesophageal, in which the stomach pushes through the hiatus and lies parallel with the esophagus.

How are they found, and how are they treated?

X rays usually can pinpoint the condition.

Sliding hiatals should be treated just like heartburn: (1) Avoid fatty foods, citric juices, garlic, onions, coffee, and alcohol; (2) eat slowly; and (3) stop smoking.

Paraesophageal hiatals, if they become inflamed, may require surgery. The operation is relatively simple, involving the use of a laparoscope, a tiny instrument that allows the surgeon to see inside the stomach. Complete recovery takes place within a couple of weeks.

What more can I do to keep a hiatal hernia benign?

Keep in mind that pressure on the stomach will accentuate the condition. Eat smaller, if more frequent, meals; avoid tight clothing; don't lie down with a full stomach.

Holiday Stress

At first glance, placing the disorder known as holiday stress in this group may seem incongruous. But it deserves inclusion for two reasons: It is one of the most common illnesses we treat, and it causes real pain.

Why do I feel increased discomfort during the holidays?

The reasons can be manifold, including too much food, too little sleep, overindulgence in alcohol, and the daunting challenge of holiday chores, as well as draining personal conflicts, dashed expectations, and poignant memories.

How can I decompress?

Take the time to identify the underlying causes of your pain. Be honest with yourself. Most cases of heightened stress spring from denial. Smoldering resentments and repressed emotions have a way of rising to the surface during the holidays. Face up to them, and put them in perspective.

Simultaneously, take care not to weaken your body. Be temperate in your eating and drinking, get enough rest, don't try to cram a week of tasks into an afternoon or evening.

How much do my sleeping and dietary habits affect my pain?

To a great degree. Partying, heavy scheduling, traveling, and new sleeping environments all contribute to a disturbed sleep, making you more vulnerable to pain.

Skipping meals to do chores, and snacking instead on nonnutrious foods, likewise impair your metabolism.

What can I do about personal conflicts?

The holidays are supposed to be a time when we're all happy. The truth, however, is that our expectations often come crashing down, causing us real anguish. The absence of some family members and friends can bring longing and grief; the presence of others can raise feelings of guilt and resentment.

How to cope? We have already suggested putting your expectations in perspective. But sometimes the rational must give way to the spiritual. In the wise words of Ruth Graham, wife of the Reverend Billy Graham, "Pray for a thick skin and a tender heart."

Why do I feel that I can't make everybody happy?

Probably because you can't. Some guests want to eat early, others late.

Some want red meat, others vegetarian fare. Some are awful, some convivial. Your efforts to accommodate everybody can, if pushed far enough, drive you over the top.

Our advice: Realize that you're only human, and enjoy the party.

Insect Bites

Most insect stings cause minor redness and swelling that last only a few hours or days.

Bites from some mosquitoes, however, can transmit malaria and encephalitis; from some ticks, Lyme disease; from some spiders and bees, intense pain and muscle spasms, developing into a condition called anaphylactic shock.

Why is swelling usually associated with insect bites?

The insect's salivary fluid is often toxic. The more powerful the toxin, the greater the swelling.

How do I ease the pain?

For ordinary bites, use cold compresses, calamine lotion, or hydrocortisone ointment.

If you find a tick, remove the insect with tweezers and show it to your doctor. In the meantime, put an ice cube over the bite.

If you think you have a bad spider or bee bite, see your doctor immediately if the initial pain worsens or you begin wheezing, become dizzy, or get a rash. You may be suffering from anaphylactic shock.

How do I avoid the problem in the first place?

Insects can be a problem almost anywhere. So ask questions. Around marshes or by the seaside, your neighbors could tell you whether the mosquitoes are just a nuisance or are carrying encephalitis. Inland, they could tell you whether deer ticks are spreading Lyme disease. Listen to what your neighbors have to say.

What other precautions should I take?

Insects are naturally drawn to warm orifices—nasal passages, ears, the mouth, genital areas—so take care to protect those areas.

Wearing proper clothing to shield your skin is also important— long pants, long-sleeved shirts, high-topped shoes, and thick socks. In the morning shake out your shoes before putting your feet in them.

Jaw Pain

The temporomandibular joint (TMJ) is the vulnerable hinge that joins the jawbone to the skull. Strains or blows that throw it out of align- ment are a major cause of jaw and facial discomfort.

How does the TMJ work?

The joint's function can be compared to using chopsticks: one stick stays fixed while the other moves up and down against it to pick up food. The upper, or maxilla, jaw remains fixed while the lower, or mandible, jaw does the moving.

But the TMJ is capable not only of opening and closing but also of moving laterally, and this flexibility is its weakness. Strong muscles in the jaw and neck can dislocate the joint, whether by chewing hard food or by grinding one's teeth. Blows to the head can cause similar damage.

Acupressure often provides some immediate relief for the pain. Using your first and second fingers, exert gentle pressure on the area above the lower-jaw hinge, just below your ears. Hold your fingers there for several seconds, then relax. Repeat the procedure up to ten times.

TMJ sufferers usually are compulsive personalities, people who drive themselves too hard. The only lasting cure, we tell them, is to (1) reexamine their lives and (2) rearrange their priorities.

Why do bad teeth hurt so much?

Teeth have nerve routes that go deep into the jaw. As a result, when a tooth decays, pain spreads over the entire facial area. Even low-level infections—such as gum disease, gingivitis, or temperature sensitivity—radiate outward. Often the pain overflows into the surrounding muscles, reinforcing the discomfort.

For temporary relief, rinse around the infection with salt water. To numb the gum, you can suck on an ice cube or rub on an over-the-counter preparation like tincture of myrrh. Ultimately, however, there's no substitute for regular visits to the dentist.

How does a bad "bite" cause jaw and facial pain?

The alignment of teeth and jaw, loosely described as one's "bite," can transmit severe pressure on the head and neck. Missing teeth, orthodontic problems, and poor bite patterns all contribute to jaw and facial pain.

Dental appliances such as plates and braces are helpful in easing the discomfort.

Does tension first manifest itself in the jaw area?

That's a fair assessment. Many people initially recognize the extent of their stress only when they find themselves clenching their jaw or gritting their teeth. Once again, our advice is deceptively simple: sit down, take several deep breaths, make a conscious effort to relax.

Joint Replacements

When do joints need to be replaced?

Such surgery is done in cases of degenerative or rheumatoid arthritis, dying blood vessels, or degenerating bone lesions.

The mechanical implant actually replaces the original joint and mimics its function but often is incapable of the original's full range of motion.

Sometimes, if the replacement fails, joint surgery must be repeated.

I thought my pain would ease immediately after joint replacement. Why has it increased?

People who have undergone the testing, preparation, medical clearance, and, ultimately, the surgical procedure itself are often surprised by postoperative discomfort. But such temporary pain is to be expected. Skin, muscle, tissue, and bone have been opened to remove the joint and insert its replacement, incurring deep trauma.

Of course, if intense or prolonged pain is felt, clinical reevaluation is necessary. Postoperative complications can include fluid accumulation, bleeding, blood clots, phlebitis, or a malaligned implant.

Even in normal cases, however, it takes time for postoperative pain and swelling to recede, for the various tissue layers to heal, for bone calluses to cushion the implant. During this period, your doctor will prescribe appropriate painkillers.

Later, when the recovery process permits, physical therapy will help you fully regain the use of your limb.

How do I protect my joint replacement?

The implant cannot be expected, any more than the original joint could, to withstand sudden impacts or unwise exertions. Blows, falls, or repetitive stress may all damage or dislodge the prosthesis.

How long will the replacement last?

That depends on the quality of the hardware. Implants are continually improving, and today's replacements last significantly longer than those of ten years ago.

Other health problems also determine how long the prosthesis remains problem-free. People with muscle spasticity or rigidity (Parkinson's disease, multiple sclerosis, spinal-cord injury) put great stress on the implant, risking dislocation.

Recurring pain after many years of feeling little or no discomfort is a sure sign that the replacement is loosening.

How bad does the pain have to be before I need an implant?

The pain must be intense, usually disabling. For hip and knee replacements, there should be a progressive loss of mobility; in hand and shoulder replacements, an ever greater loss of function.

Before opting for surgery, keep in mind that painful joint conditions have other solutions, including braces, oral medications, and injections into the joint. Only when these have failed should surgery be considered.

Which is more harmful to the implant, trauma or repetitive stress?

Trauma is, of course, a single occurrence; the resulting harm is immediate and easily identified.

A more insidious problem is repetitive stress, whereby patients often do not realize the damage they are inflicting. Careless, ill-considered pressures, building up year after year, greatly shorten the implant's life.

Mononucleosis

Why is mononucleosis called the "kissing disease"?

Because the virus that causes the condition (named the Epstein-Barr virus, after its British discoverers) is commonly spread through saliva.

What are the symptoms?

Fever, fatigue, sore throat, and swollen lymph nodes in the neck.

Is mononucleosis difficult to diagnose?

Its symptoms are quite similar to those of the flu and strep throat, but a blood test can quickly verify the condition.

How long does mono last, and how is it treated?

The acute stage lasts about two weeks, and it's not unusual for complete recovery to take two months.

Bed rest is prescribed for at least the first few weeks, along with drugs like acetaminophen for the fever and prednisone for the sore throat. Because the virus may weaken the spleen, posing the possibility of rupturing it, patients are cautioned against heavy lifting and similar abdominal strain.

How can I help myself recover?

Take frequent naps, drink plenty of liquids, keep your energy level high with small snacks, gargle with warm salt water, and stimulate your kidneys by massaging your lower back several times a day.

Are there alternative medicines and therapies?

Herbal teas containing echinacea may reduce mono's infectious aspects, while St.-John's-wort may relieve the depression many patients feel during the lengthy recuperation period.

Reducing stress, and the toll it takes on the body's immune system, is extremely important. Patients should be encouraged to master such techniques as biofeedback, guided imagery, or quiet meditation.

Mouth Sores

What are canker sores, and what causes them?

They're small white spots that appear inside the lips and mouth. We don't really know what causes them, but some experts attribute them to stress.

What treatment exists?

The sores last a week to ten days and usually heal themselves. Meanwhile, anesthetics such as lidocaine can be applied or used as mouthwash.

What are cold sores?

Cold sores, or fever blisters, are brought on by the herpes simplex virus and can appear anywhere in the mouth, but always on the gums. Since the disease is viral, it never leaves the body but rather just goes into remission between flare-ups.

And the treatment?

Again, lidocaine will ease the pain. Zovirax, an antiviral drug, can be used in capsule or ointment form to speed the healing. Attacks last at least a week.

Multiple Sclerosis (MS)

Multiple sclerosis, a disease of the central nervous system, attacks and partially destroys the myelin sheath, the protective substance around the nerves. Once the myelin disintegrates, the nerves in effect short-circuit. Symptoms include spasticity or tremors in the limbs, a loss of balance, visual problems, and incontinence. MS affects twice as many women as men.

What causes MS?

Nobody really knows, but many clinicians feel that it may arise from a weakness in the immune system. Attacks come and go as the myelin sheath becomes inflamed and then heals itself. Once the sheath is gone, however, the condition becomes permanent.

Is the latest research encouraging insofar as a possible cure is concerned?

Scientists who recently analyzed nervous-system brain tissue from patients suffering acute attacks of multiple sclerosis think the disease may result from a combination of factors—ranging from failures in the immune system to viruses to toxins.

This would help explain the striking differences in symptoms among sufferers, some having cycles of relapse and recovery and some steadily deteriorating. A study in the *Annals of Neurology* claims to have found four separate patterns of multiple-sclerosis damage in the brain's nerve sheath.

Once the researchers fully interpret these patterns, they hope to use them to develop targeted medications for the disease.

What do you mean by spasticity in the limbs?

The nerve lesions cause an uncontrolled reflex that results in spastic, or tightly contracted, muscles. If the limb affected is not moved regularly, either actively or passively, it becomes permanently contracted.

Spasticity is sometimes relieved with corticosteroids and muscle relaxants, physical therapy, or a range of motion exercises. In severe cases, invasive procedures like surgical blocks (surgical releases of the muscles/tendons) or nerve blocks (chemical injections) may be needed.

How does the lack of movement in the limbs affect MS sufferers?

Contracted muscles affect the position of arms and legs, keeping the patient from sitting or standing comfortably. Over time even simple articles of clothing become more and more difficult to put on and take off. Practicing proper hygiene becomes increasingly troublesome. Restful sleep is impossible. Open ulcers may develop, accentuating the pain.

Are MS sufferers permanently fatigued?

Yes, for all of the above reasons.

What psychological problems are associated with MS?

Depression, mood swings, irritability, and thoughts of suicide are all common and all lower the patient's ability to tolerate pain. Psychotherapy is required as much as physical therapy.

Neck Pain

This condition can begin as a spinal nerve irritation or an aching of the musculature surrounding the neck, shoulders, and lower skull. As it increases, neck pain can "spread," causing upper-shoulder, arm, and headache discomfort.

What does a soft collar accomplish?

Most people have seen surgical, or soft, collars and wondered about their use. Such collars offer almost no cervical support but provide comfort to the neck and its muscles. Simultaneously, they remind the wearer to limit and reduce stress on the cervical vertebrae.

How does neck pain generally develop, and how can it be eased?

Emotional stress often causes muscular tension, bringing about stiffness and aching in the cervical region. We teach patients how to relax and ease the tension. Ultimately, we want them to identify and eliminate the source of their stress before they get locked into a chronic condition.

Where do the nerves in the neck lead?

The nerves that originate in the cervical spine pass through outlets, or "windows," and are distributed to various sites in the upper body. These sites include the back of the head, jaws, upper shoulders, arms, and hands.

Why does it feel good to rotate my head and "crack" my neck?

Some people perceive popping and cracking sounds when they rotate their heads. Nobody really knows whether the origin of these sounds is harmful or beneficial. They may be caused by ligaments and tendons rubbing over the vertebrae or by subtle displacements within the spinal column. Or they may result from the release of nitrogen or other gasses within the cervical vertebrae, thereby creating a change in pressure.

What kind of diagnostic tools are used in treating neck pain?

Basically the same tests that are used for lower-back pain: X rays, CAT scans, and MRIs.

Is the spine in my neck the same as the one in my lower back?

The spinal column begins beneath the skull and runs to the coccyx, or tailbone. The nerves are housed within the bony vertebrae. The spine's architecture varies, depending on its function. The lumbar, or lower-back, vertebrae are bigger and stronger; the neck, or cervical, vertebrae are smaller and have greater rotational qualities.

All the vertebrae are cushioned by discs made of cartilage. When a disc ruptures, or herniates, it bulges outward, often irritating nearby nerves. While the lower back is much more vulnerable to disc herniation, the condition also occurs in the neck area.

When is surgery indicated?

For any kind of pain originating in the vertebrae, surgery should be the therapy of last resort. It should be considered only if there is constant and irreversible pain, neuromuscular impairment, and bladder and bowel degeneration.

What kind of exercises prevent and relieve neck pain?

Here are two:

1. From a standing position, feet together, bend forward at the waist, exhaling and dropping your head toward the floor. Grasp your elbows, inhale, hold your breath for several seconds, release your breath, stand upright. Do ten repetitions, gradually increasing to twenty-five.

2. Sit upright on a chair or stool. Slowly lift and lower one shoulder, then the other, then both shoulders together. Do ten repetitions, building up to twenty-five.

Neuralgia

Neuralgia is nerve pain resulting from inflammation or pressure on the nerve. It is usually sharp and burning, occurs on only one side of the body, and can be intermittent or continuous.

What kinds of neuralgia are there?

The principal types are (1) trigeminal, or facial, neuralgia; (2) sciatica, which occurs in the lower back and legs; and (3) postherpetic neuralgia, which strikes almost anywhere and is associated with the herpes rash called shingles.

What medications are prescribed?

Generally speaking, analgesics and sedatives to ease the pain, and corticosteroids to reduce inflammation. For facial neuralgia, anticonvulsant drugs can be beneficial; for shingles, Zovirax ointment.

What alternative therapies for neuralgia are there?

The best emphasize relaxation: the Alexander method, which relieves pressure by teaching proper posture; deep massage, which loosens the tissues; and acupuncture, which increases circulation to the nerves, causing pain reduction.

Why does nerve pain linger?

The initial damage to the nerve may have been resolved, but it continues to send out "distress" signals. Neuralgia is like an on/off switch stuck in the on position. Pain can persist for months or years.

Osteoporosis

Osteoporosis is the loss of bone mass, making the bones porous and more brittle and increasing the likelihood of fractures. Calcium, the skeleton's hardening element, begins to decline in our middle years, so the disease is, to some degree, part of the aging process. Symptoms include backaches and stooped posture.

Who is at risk?

Four out of every five sufferers are women, most in the years after menopause, when their calcium decline intensifies. Slim, fine-boned, fair-complected women are most at risk, as are those who miss their periods because of heavy exercise (amenorrhea) or nutritional deprivation (anorexia).

What other causes contribute to loss of bone mass?

Underlying diseases, poor nutrition in general, excessive use of caffeine and alcohol, and immobilization in a cast or brace.

So it's "thinning" of the bones that makes falls more serious for the elderly?

That's correct. A young person falls and does nothing worse than bruise some soft tissue. An elderly person takes the same tumble and fractures a hip.

Why does osteoporosis make my bones "hurt"?

You are experiencing chronic skeletal pain, possibly as a result of multiple minifractures. These are hairline breaks in the bone, not serious enough to require a cast but sufficient to make you thoroughly uncomfortable. If they're in the spine, they're responsible for stooped posture.

Are some parts of the body more vulnerable than others?

Fractures can occur just about anywhere—shoulders, wrists, hips, or ankles. The disease affects the entire skeleton, so no one bone or joint is more at risk than others.

How important is calcium in my diet?

Adequate calcium intake for adults should be about 1–1.5 grams daily. But many calcium-rich foods are high in fat content, which can bring on other health problems. Instead, ingest low-fat milk and yogurt, as well as leafy green vegetables. Avoid red meats and soft drinks, which make it difficult for the body to absorb calcium.

Supplements, available in vitamin shops and drugstores, can be helpful as long as they are not taken to excess.

How is the onset of osteoporosis detected?

The best test for early detection is with computerized tomography, which is a computer-enhanced X ray. Ordinary X rays don't spot bone loss until it's relatively advanced.

How can I keep osteoporosis in check?

For postmenopausal women, medication therapy calls for hormone replacement. If you stop taking the hormones, however, the loss of bone mass resumes.

For everyone, men and women, the best natural therapy is pursuing a long-term exercise program—half an hour to an hour, three to five times a week. Running, fast walking, tennis, and aerobics are beneficial because they put body weight on the skeletal structure. It's a truism: to keep bones from weakening, you must put calculated stress on them.

Parkinson's Disease

This degenerative disease of the nervous system begins with minor shaking, say, in a limb, then progressively worsens, affecting posture, balance, coordination, speech, and swallowing.

What causes Parkinson's?

Dopamine (one of the two substances in the brain that regulate neural transmissions) loses its potency, creating a chemical imbalance that affects bodily functions.

What kind of functions?

Here are some examples:

- Bradykinesia, or slowed movements, typically noticeable in hand and arm motions and in walking.

- Akinesia, or the inability to initiate a desired movement. The will is present, but the limbs do not react.

- Low phonation, or low-volume speech and low-level breath control. The patient has difficulty in coughing or in clearing pulmonary secretions.

- Festenating gait, or a forwardly propelled, head-first, impulsive manner of walking.

- Monotonous, or droning, speech patterns.

- Muscle rigidity, or cogwheeling, ratchetlike movements of the limbs.

Is Parkinson's a painful syndrome?

Not especially. But the resulting limb contractions and postural deformities do lead to chronic, low-level discomfort.

Patients are, of course, quite likely to suffer falls, and all such injuries should be carefully evaluated.

How are Parkinson's symptoms treated?

Various medications, such as levadopa, serve as a substitute for the brain's natural dopamine and can be quite effective. In extreme cases, neurosurgery is performed.

Physical therapy calls for postural retraining to restore the patient's balance while walking, standing, and sitting. The use of seating inserts, proper bed and bathroom equipment, and other items further the rehabilitation process.

Can you be more specific about a drug program to treat Parkinson's?

Once again, this is a matter on which the patient and the physician must confer. Each case is unique. Drugs must be introduced in the proper sequence, and possible side effects must be carefully observed. The extent of the disease and the possibility of multiple medications further complicate the equation.

Your doctor should consider your case a work in progress, listen to your reports of positive and negative reactions to the drugs, and respond accordingly.

What are the latest experimental findings on the Parkinson's front?

Scientists at the Robert Wood Johnson Medical School in Piscataway, New Jersey, have removed cells from the bone marrow of rats—and humans—that normally would have developed into tendon, cartilage, and bone and have grown them in laboratory dishes. By adding an antioxidant, beta-mercaptoethanol, to the marrow cells, the researchers converted them into nerve cells, raising the possibility that a new source of replacement cells might be in the offing to treat brain diseases like Parkinson's and Alzheimer's.

While the findings are still in the experimental stage, the results thus far are encouraging. Dr. Ira Black, chairman of the Department of Neuroscience and Cell Biology at the Johnson facility, stated that he and his colleagues had an 80 percent success rate in converting the marrow cells into nerve cells. Going a step further, they then transplanted the rat nerve cells into the brains and spinal cords of live rats, thus far without negative side effects.

Plant Allergies

Can contact with plants cause pain?

Certain plants contain allergens and toxins that result in painful dermatitis and itching. Poison ivy, poison oak, and poison sumac are common examples. Plants having toxin-laden spurs, such as cactus and burrs, cause similar reactions.

What are some remedies?

For the rash, cool compresses and over-the-counter medications, like calamine lotion and hydrocortisone ointment, and homemade pastes— oatmeal and water, or baking soda and water—are beneficial.

If the itch is particularly bad, put aside the cool compresses and bathe the area in very hot water. This will temporarily heighten the itch, then give you two or three hours of relief.

Toxins are easily spread by rubbing. Take care to avoid their coming into contact with the eyes and face.

What preventive steps can I take?

Familiarity with the shape, color, and leaf appearance of toxic plants is essential and relatively easy to achieve. All sorts of nature books and pamphlets are available.

Gardeners in particular should use gloves and wear forearm protection.

Postsurgical Pain

Doctors usually inform patients about the risks and associated procedural steps of surgery, but sometimes they don't spell out what patients can expect in its aftermath. This is a serious mistake, because the postsurgical period, and the patient's reaction to it, can determine whether the operation is a success.

So patients in the postoperative period can to some degree undermine the surgery?

Yes, if they react in a depressed and negative manner to the realities of internal bleeding, restricted mobility, fluid accumulation and drainage, and possible infection.

Patients should be informed that surgery often requires deep incisions, with corresponding damage to surrounding tissue and bone. They should be told that the procedure may bring on temporary discomfort, but lasting relief. Otherwise, through fear or lack of knowledge, they may slow or even subvert the healing process.

Naturally, all manner of painkilling medications are available, in variable combinations and variable dosages, to mitigate the discomfort. Good doctors will prescribe relief according to each individual's needs.

How long does postoperative pain last?

It varies from procedure to procedure and from person to person. But surgeons can make informed estimates by racheting the average experience up or down depending on one's age and overall physical condition.

Prolonged pain is often experienced by people with preexisting conditions or poor underlying health.

Will my scar always look like that?

Patients often are frightened the first time they see their scar. The sutures, redness, and edema around the incision make a disturbing sight. But once the sutures are removed (usually ten days to a few weeks after surgery) and the redness and swelling disappear, the scar becomes far less alarming.

Will it hurt when the stitches come out?

You're not alone in fearing that the removal of surgical stitches or staples will be a painful process. But there is little discomfort—perhaps a pinching feeling.

Admittedly, some people do have scar sensitivity. But for most, the pain is associated more with anticipation than actuality. Doctors should discuss the procedure with patients and help them relax.

How can I reduce the edema?

Immediate postsurgical swelling is relieved by elevating the affected area and, to restore the circulation of fluid, flexing the muscles in the limbs. Sometimes compressive dressings are helpful.

After a patient's discharge, specific therapy is tailored to the individual. Postmastectomy recovery, for instance, calls for massage, exercising the arms, and using compressive garments.

Why is my scar so sensitive?

Some people are more sensitive than others to the tissue growth, directly under the scar, that occurs during healing. Light massage generally helps.

In most cases, this syndrome resolves itself with time.

Pregnancy and Childbirth

Is pain during pregnancy normal?

Various levels of discomfort may be expected during pregnancy—including nausea, aching muscles, abdominal and back pain, and leg and hand edema—as the body hormonally and physically reacts to the growing fetus.

Intense or persistent pain is not normal, however, and requires clinical evaluation.

You should visit your doctor regularly—to ensure the healthy development of the fetus, your present and future health, and a safe delivery.

Will my pain be variable?

Your discomfort usually changes as your pregnancy advances.

The first trimester may bring you minor aches, nausea, increased urination, and a sense of malaise; the second trimester, weight gain and swelling of the extremities, abdominal and back pain, and constipation; the third trimester, a worsening of all these symptoms.

You should understand, however, that you can do much to lessen your discomfort.

Generally speaking, what steps can I take?

Here are some suggestions:

- **Clothing:** Wear loose-fitting attire and sensible shoes. If necessary, wear a support bra for enlarged breasts and support hose for edema.

- **Diet:** Observe a nonfatty, high-fiber diet that will both keep your weight under control and facilitate bowel movements.

Drink plenty of water, avoid painkillers, and check with your doctor before taking any medications.

- **Lifestyle:** Elevate your legs as much as possible to reduce edema, and avoid prolonged standing. Get plenty of sleep.

- **Exercise:** Ask your doctor for simple exercises that will lessen abdominal and back pain and will strengthen the uterus.

When I gain weight during pregnancy, where is my body most affected?

Significant weight gain leads to pelvic and lumbar stresses, with the attendant pain, and varicosity and edema in the legs.

Will my age add to my discomfort?

More mature women, in part because they may have preexisting health problems, usually require closer monitoring than younger ones.

They should report all such problems to their obstetricians at the onset of prenatal care.

I desperately want a child, but I fear the pain involved. How can I overcome my qualms?

There are many myths about the travails of pregnancy and childbirth, and you owe it to yourself to dispel them.

Start by ignoring the dire warnings from uninformed sources. Choose a knowledgeable obstetrician and let the doctor allay your fears. Expand your confidence by reading pamphlets and books on the subject and participate in programs designed to reduce discomfort before, during, and after delivery.

Finally, tone up both your body and your mind. Physically, pursue a nutritious diet, avoid toxins, lose weight if necessary, and exercise appropriately. Mentally, pursue such relaxation techniques as meditation, guided imagery, and hypnotherapy.

What role does ultrasound play in indicating the health of the fetus?

Ultrasound machines have revolutionized prenatal monitoring. Not only can doctors and parents-to-be look at the fetus's beating heart and moving hands and feet, but physicians can to a large degree determine its health. They do so by measuring the fetus's overall length, the length of the thighbone, the circumference of the head and abdomen, the composition of the kidney and bladder, and the strength of the heart chambers.

In the first trimester these scans are used to determine fetal age by measuring crown–rump length and head circumference. In the second trimester doctors measure abdominal circumference and check out the fetus's organs. Between seventeen and nineteen weeks of gestation, for instance, the thighbone is examined to evaluate the likelihood of Down's syndrome.

Ultrasound's importance, however, should not be stressed to the point of regarding it as omnipotent. Dr. Roy Filly, professor of radiology at the University of California at San Francisco School of Medicine, recently decried its overuse. "From my standpoint," he wrote in the *Journal of Ultrasound in Medicine*, "the identification of 'abnormalities' in low-risk women has crossed the line of 'more harm than good.' We put at least ten percent of all pregnant women with perfectly normal fetuses through a good deal of worry."

Why do many women experience morning sickness in the early months of pregnancy?

First of all, understand that the term *morning sickness* is a misnomer. Pregnant women can experience nausea and vomiting at any time during the day.

Understand further that such nausea, in the past at least, was nature's way of helping pregnant women avoid such foods as meat, fish, poultry, and eggs. Before the advent of refrigeration, these were the products most likely to harbor toxic organisms that could damage the fetus or even bring on a miscarriage.

Studies show that even today women who suffer morning sickness symptoms are far less likely to have miscarriages or stillbirths than those who are symptom-free.

What problems can be expected during postpartum recovery?

General fatigue, muscle aches, and pelvic discomfort are not uncommon. To relieve these symptoms, light exercise—under the direction of the obstetrician—is usually beneficial.

Similarly, exercise is a key factor in overcoming postpartum depression, taking the individual out of herself and into the physical world.

I may need a cesarean section. What pain will I encounter?

You will need additional time to heal your surgical wounds and scars, so you should expect a longer postpartum recovery period. With proper treatment, however, you should be confident that your pain can be mitigated and your stomach muscles restored.

Is breast-feeding painful?

Women who breast-feed may experience discomfort from breast-milk engorgement or from nipple dryness and cracking. The use of breast pumps, as well as the use of topical ointments on the nipples, can lessen these problems significantly.

Premenstrual Syndrome (PMS)

Is PMS a syndrome or a myth?

It's very much a physical syndrome and is experienced, either regularly or infrequently, by most women. Symptoms can be mild or strong and include headaches, insomnia, anxiety, depression, and irritability, as well as water retention, muscle aches, acne, hot flashes, and bowel and urinary irregularities.

Some people worry that the reality of PMS, which usually strikes about a week before menstruation, is used to put down women, minimizing the gains they have made in the workplace. We feel that such worry is unfounded. The symptoms, while distressing, are for most women far from disabling.

Is the PMS experience the same for all women?

No, it differs from person to person. Age, weight, body type, diet, emotional outlook, and personality may all affect the severity of the symptoms, as may individual pain tolerance—but no definitive study exists.

How do I know whether PMS is causing some of the symptoms you mention, or whether some other illness is?

You should seek regular gynecological care. Chances are that your gynecologist will have you keep a diary to see when the symptoms come and go. That process should tell you whether your problems are part of your menstrual cycle.

The women who experience intense PMS symptoms are a minority, we emphasize, but they require close clinical evaluation. More grievous problems, such as uterine fibroids, ovarian cysts, and gynecological tumors, produce similar symptoms.

Don't some men use PMS to denigrate women?

Unfortunately, yes. But their efforts are misguided and, sometimes, even misogynistic. Women have normal emotional reactions, and to say that these responses are purely hormonal in nature is an exercise in negativity. Male and female interaction is strongest when there is open, positive communication.

How is PMS treated professionally?

Through hormone therapy, usually estrogen or progesterone, that is administered locally or through injections. Some women experience severe side effects from the hormones, however, and turn to other remedies.

Like what?

- Chamomile or other herbal tea, warm baths, and mild diuretics all lessen irritability and anxiety.

- Yoga and light exercise, which release more endorphins in the brain, are helpful in easing aches and pains.

- Eat lightly (perhaps five or six snacks rather than three meals) in the week before your period, avoid caffeine and alcohol, get enough sleep.

How can I tell the difference between anxiety and PMS?

The symptoms admittedly can be quite similar. But keeping the menstrual diary we mentioned earlier will help you pinpoint the *source* of your anxiety. If you find that it coincides with your cycle, you'll know it's PMS-associated.

Prostate Pain

What is the prostate?

It is the small gland at the base of the bladder that surrounds part of the urethra, the tube that carries urine and sperm out of the body through the penis.

Are there different kinds of prostate discomfort?

Primarily, there are two—one coming from an enlarged prostate, the other from a bacterial infection.

Prostate enlargement, which affects fully half of all men over fifty, pinches the urethra and can cause the bladder's not being able to empty completely, dribbling, and recurring urges to urinate—particularly at night.

The bacterial infection, called prostatitis, is either acute or chronic and can cause severe pain in the penile and anal areas, chills and fever, more pronounced urinary difficulties, and sexual dysfunction.

How do doctors identify prostate problems?

If the doctor suspects enlargement, he puts his finger into the rectum and feels the extent of the gland's growth.

If he suspects prostatitis, he orders a blood test and follows up with a tactile examination of the gland.

Do these conditions often lead to prostate cancer?

There's no proven link, although many of the symptoms are similar. Prostate cancer generally is spotted when the doctor notes that the enlarged prostate is not smooth but studded with nodules. Subsequently, a biopsy can determine whether they are benign or malignant.

Even if cancer is discovered, surgery or similar radical treatment is not always necessary. The nodules may be confined to a small area or be only mildly malignant, meaning that they would not be life-threatening for some time. Particularly if the patient is elderly, the doctor may recommend adopting a wait-and-see approach.

What therapies exist for prostate enlargement and prostatitis?

Enlargement problems are helped by such drugs as terazosin, which relaxes the bladder muscles, or by finasteride, which shrinks the prostate itself. Minor surgery can be performed without cutting but under anesthesia by passing an instrument up the penis to clear a urinary path through the gland. The procedure, called a transurethral resection, is highly effective, but in one out of every ten cases can result in complications like incontinence or impotence.

Prostatitis symptoms usually are treated with antibiotics and nonsteroidal anti-inflammatory drugs (NSAIDs). Drinking plenty of water and taking stool softeners also are beneficial.

Are there alternative therapies?

Symptoms of prostate enlargement may be helped by saw palmetto extract and by various yoga exercises performed while lying on the stomach, which are meant to stimulate the pelvis.

Chronic prostatitis may benefit from such herbs as pipsissewa and from foods rich in zinc, such as wheat bran, oatmeal, and sunflower seeds.

Psoriasis

Red patches on the skin, accompanied by white scales, denote psoriasis. The disease can spread all over the body but tends to concentrate on the scalp, elbows, knees, and legs.

What causes it?

The best guess is emotional stress, which weakens the immune system and allows skin cells to multiply abnormally.

Who gets psoriasis?

Mostly fair-skinned people.

How is it treated?

The disease responds well to the same medications that help dermatitis—vitamin D cream, corticosteroids, and coal tars.

Ultraviolet light therapy under medical supervision is also beneficial, particularly if the scaling is so widespread that applying salve becomes a chore.

What else can I do?

- If you live in a warm climate, expose your skin to sunlight frequently. (Use the appropriate sunscreens, of course, so you don't risk skin cancer.)

- To alleviate stress, set aside part of each day for meditation, spiritual reflection, or light exercise.

- Fish oil capsules may help lubricate your skin.

- Avoid ingesting citrus fruits, and drink alcohol sparingly.

Pulmonary Diseases (asthma, bronchitis, emphysema)

These diseases occur when the lungs' airways become constricted and mucus buildup causes breathing problems. Asthma attacks, which are triggered by allergies or stress, are episodic in nature and can be accompanied by gasping or wheezing. Acute bronchitis, which is usually brought on by a viral infection, is nonetheless treated with antibiotics because of collateral bacterial infection, and symptoms include a hacking cough and phlegm. Chronic bronchitis, on the other hand, results from cigarette smoking or long-term exposure to irritants in the air. Emphysema, a progressive pulmonary disease, likewise evolves from continual exposure to irritants and can be fatal.

Why does my chest hurt in chronic lung complaints?

Because your lungs are not functioning properly, ancillary muscles attempt to compensate. Puffing, wheezing, coughing, gasping, or simply expelling air—these are all adaptive measures to help you breathe. This "compensation" puts a significant, and painful, strain on the chest, even up to the neck and vocal cords.

Why am I coughing?

Coughing is the abdominal muscles clearing excessive pulmonary secretions, or mucus, and facilitating breathing. Such secretions encourage congestion, pneumonia, even abscesses.

The price you pay for prolonged coughing is irritation in your chest and abdomen, frustration, and eventually exhaustion.

How do my emotions add to my discomfort?

Chronic lung conditions bring on repeated attacks, so you're in a permanent state of anxiety. When an attack does occur, your anxiety turns to panic, heightening your sense of pain.

What are some solutions for chronic lung problems?

Asthma sufferers, of course, should try to identify and avoid their allergies. Chronic bronchitis and emphysema sufferers should give up smoking (and if the workplace is causing their problems, change their jobs).

To clear up mucus, suctioning can be effective, as well as medications such as bronchodilators.

In therapy sessions, patients are taught improved techniques for adaptive breathing. The aim is to slow the respiratory rate, increase cough efficiency, and lower vocal-cord strain. Spirometers, gadgets that require patients to suck on a tube to raise a small ball in the air, can be useful in this regard.

What are the latest medications for asthma relief?

Scientists are experimenting with a treatment called anti-IgE, short for immunoglobulin E, one of the antibodies that fight foreign intruders in the body. IgE is shaped like an inverted letter Y, two tails hanging freely and the third tail attached to the cells. When an allergen enters the body, it irritates the tails and causes them to spew the substances that distress the eyes and clog the bronchial tubes. The anti-IgE shots block the IgE antibody at the cell level, stopping the spread of the irritants at the source.

While anti-IgE could have a major impact on asthma sufferers, more tests have to be done before its effectiveness can be truly established.

Raynaud's Syndrome

What is this disease?

Raynaud's syndrome, named for the French doctor who first discovered the condition, is a circulatory problem. The blood vessels in the extremities, primarily the hands and feet, overreact to relatively mild drops in temperature. Numbness affects the fingers and toes, which turn first white, then blue.

The syndrome can also be caused by stress.

Who gets it?

Eighty percent of sufferers are young women.

What are the causes?

It's pretty much a guessing game. Possibilities include rheumatoid arthritis, atherosclerosis, and damage to the nerve endings.

How is Raynaud's treated?

Cacium channel blockers like nifedipine, which dilate the arteries, are sometimes prescribed for severe cases.

Most people cope with the disease themselves, however, by exercising, trying to stay out of the cold, and taking precautions when they must go outdoors.

Here are some tips:

- Avoid smoking, which constricts the blood vessels.

- Fish oil, taken in capsule form, may stimulate circulation.

- Dress in loose layers, so you can easily adjust to the temperature.

- Consider using chemical "warmers" in your mittens and shoes.

Sciatica

What are the symptoms of sciatica?
Pain, either sporadic or continuous, radiates through your buttock, thigh, and lower leg.

Why is it happening?
Your sciatic nerve, which extends the length of your leg, is feeling irritation, perhaps from a damaged vertebrae or a slipped disc, perhaps from osteoarthritis.

Can the exact point of the irritation be found?
Usually, through X rays, MRIs, and computerized tomography (CT) scans.

How is sciatica treated?
Painkillers, anti-inflammatories, or corticosteroids may be prescribed. Such medications, together with rest and restricting one's movements, generally alleviate the irritation.

What can I do to help myself?
- Learn the correct way to sit, walk, and stand. The so-called Alexander technique, a training program, is quite helpful in this regard.

- During attacks, apply ice packs for at least thirty minutes half a dozen times a day. Sleep on a firm mattress, on your back, with a pillow under your knees.

Scoliosis

What is scoliosis?

It's an abnormal, sideways curvature of the spine, producing a dull, chronic pain. Most often one shoulder is forced higher than the other, while the opposite hip is pushed out as the spine evolves into an S shape.

In some cases, the rib cage can become twisted, putting adverse strain on the heart and lungs.

Who are most affected?

Adolescent boys and girls, although the disease is more serious in the latter.

Skeletal maturity occurs at thirteen or fourteen; therefore, the scoliosis curve is most responsive to correction before that age.

Can the disease strike people in middle age?

Some adults get scoliosis as a result of having diseases of the nervous system, such as cerebral palsy and multiple sclerosis. Other cases stem from trauma, such as a spinal fracture.

How is scoliosis treated?

Through exercise, orthopedic braces, and surgery, depending on how far the disease has progressed. Each patient presents a different challenge.

Exercises aimed at strengthening and simultaneously limbering the back and torso are the preferred way of tackling the problem, but sometimes the individual's condition, initially at least, precludes this solution. A torso brace is then prescribed, and perhaps posture-aiding chairs and beds as well. Therapists recognize that overusing the brace has a downside, however, ultimately weakening muscles and impairing breathing. As soon as the patient is sufficiently improved, therefore, exercise programs are instituted.

In extreme cases, metal rods are inserted surgically along the spine, arresting and correcting its curvature.

Are there secondary therapies?

TENS (transcutaneous electrical nerve stimulation) reduces the pain, and this small, portable machine can be used anywhere in the home. Hot packs are another option.

Medications include painkillers and anti-inflammatories.

Sexually Transmitted Diseases (gonorrhea, chlamydia, chancroid, syphilis, genital herpes, genital warts, AIDS, hepatitis B)

Are these diseases always transmitted through sexual intercourse?

They usually result from genital, oral, or anal intercourse with an infected partner but can be spread by kisses, contaminated hypodermic needles or blood transfusions, or tainted food or water.

Do sexually transmitted diseases (STDs) fall into distinct categories?

Diseases such as gonorrhea, chlamydia, chancroid, and syphilis are bacterial in origin; genital herpes, genital warts, AIDS, and hepatitis B are viral. The bacteria and viruses, microscopic in size, enter the body through the mucous membranes or cuts in the skin.

Syphilis is the most serious of these conditions; genital herpes, the most common.

What are the symptoms of bacterial STDs?

- **Gonorrhea and chlamydia:** Men usually suffer abdominal discomfort, painful urination, and a discharge of pus from the penis within days after infection. Most women are symptom-free, but those who engage in anal intercourse with infected men, or in oral sex, can develop painful rectum or throat problems.

- **Chancroid:** Blisters or ulcers occur around the genitals or anus.

- **Syphilis:** The untreated disease goes through three stages. First, within a week or two, a painless sore appears on the penis or vagina and then goes away. Next, weeks or months later, a skin rash makes its appearance and likewise becomes latent. Lastly, years later, the disease can recur, with drastic consequences.

How are these conditions diagnosed?

Through routine physicals, laboratory analysis of the pus, or blood tests.

What therapies exist?

Gonorrhea, chlamydia, and chancroid respond to such antibiotics as erythromycin and tetracycline, usually over seven to ten days. Syphilis, in all its stages, responds most often to penicillin.

Left untreated, what damage do these diseases inflict?

Gonorrhea can spread from a pregnant woman to the fetus during birth, causing the child's blindness. Chlamydia can affect the fallopian tubes, resulting in infertility. Syphilis, in its last stage, can lead to heart failure, blindness, or insanity.

What are the symptoms of viral STDs?

- **Genital herpes:** Both men and women suffer recurring outbreaks of itchy, watery blisters around the penis and vagina, accompanied by flulike symptoms and painful urination.

- **Genital warts:** Painless but contagious grayish growths occur in the genital or anal areas.

- **AIDS and hepatitis B:** These diseases are discussed in their own sections in this book.

How are the conditions treated?

Genital herpes cannot be cured, but antiviral drugs like acyclovir can make outbreaks shorter and less frequent.

Genital warts can be removed through laser therapy, freezing, or minor surgery.

If either partner is having an attack of genital herpes, can they still have sex?

No, they should abstain. Even when the disease is in remission, the male partner should use a condom.

Shin Splints

What are shin splints?

They're muscle tears in the lower leg. Pain may be felt in the muscles running along the front and outer part of the shinbone, or tibia, or the back and inner part.

What causes them?

Repeated stress on the leg. If your pain is in the front and outer part, you may be doing too much running or jogging. Your shin muscles, which pull the foot up, are being torn by your stronger calf muscles, which pull the heel down.

If your pain is in the back and inner part of the leg, you may be running on banked surfaces. You're rolling your ankle inward, stressing a different group of shin muscles.

How are shin splints treated?

Primarily through rest, ice, compression, and elevation—the acronym RICE. Rest gives the body the chance to heal itself; ice reduces swelling; compression with elastic bandages restricts swelling; elevation drains accumulated fluids.

Over-the-counter drugs like ibuprofen reduce the pain and inflammation.

What preventive measures can I take?

- Do stretching exercises to make your leg muscles supple before running or jogging.

- Wear athletic shoes that give you proper arch, heel, and ankle support.

Sinusitis

How does sinusitis happen?

The sinuses, four groupings of hollow cavities in the area around the nose, produce mucus that, in effect, cleans the air we breathe. If the sinuses become inflamed, however, the mucus does not drain properly and the cavities fill up, becoming a breeding ground for infection.

Why do the sinuses become irritated?

Usually because of a virus, such as the common cold. But the condition can also be caused by bacterial, fungal, or allergic agents.

What are the symptoms?

Pain around the eyes and nose, the inability to breathe through the nose, postnasal drip, and facial swelling.

How is sinusitis diagnosed?

Often in a routine examination, but deep infections may require a computerized tomography (CT) scan.

How is it treated?

Mainly through various antibiotics administered over a week or two for acute cases, longer for chronic ones.

Decongestants such as pseudoephedrine are also beneficial. Antihistamines are counterproductive, since they thicken the mucus, impeding the draining process.

Should antibiotics always be administered for sinusitis?

Some sinus problems should not be treated with antibiotics. Those caused exclusively by viruses or allergic agents will not benefit from such medications. Your doctor is the best judge of the drug you should receive.

Sprains and Tendinitis

What tissues are affected by strains and tendinitis?

Sprains are injuries to the ligaments, the fibrous tissue that connects the bones at the joints. Tendinitis, as the name implies, is damage to the tendons, the tissue that connects the muscles to the bones.

Who are more likely to get these injuries?

Sprains are more apt to occur among people who are overweight, out of shape, or engaging in unfamiliar athletic activity. Tendinitis most often results from repetitive stress.

How can I help these conditions heal?

Both injuries usually respond within weeks to the RICE regimen— rest, ice, compression, and elevation. Aspirin or ibuprofen helps relieve the pain. In some cases, however, severe ligament sprains require surgery.

Tendinitis sufferers, once the original damage is in remission, will benefit from physical-therapy programs to strengthen the muscle groups in the affected areas.

Strep Throat and Tonsillitis

What is a strep throat, and what causes it?

It's an infection caused by the common bacterium *Streptococcus pyogenes,* which lies dormant in the throat for weeks or months, only to flare up when the immune system is impaired by stress or exhaustion.

What are the symptoms?

Severe pain while swallowing, swollen lymph glands in the neck, and fever.

Can strep throat be quickly identified, and how is it treated?

The disease can be verified within minutes, right in the doctor's office. Antibiotics, probably penicillin or erythromycin, cure strep in about a week, with remission beginning in about thirty-six hours. Even quicker immediate relief can be obtained by using medicated throat sprays or by gargling with warm water.

How does tonsillitis differ from strep throat?

Though the symptoms are much the same, tonsillitis generally affects children. The tonsils are nodes of lymph tissue in the throat that play a major role in helping youngsters fight disease. Sometimes, however, the nodes themselves develop infections, becoming painful and swollen or even abcessing.

How is tonsillitis treated?

Similarly to strep throat, with antibiotics, sprays, and gargling.

How often are the tonsils surgically removed?

A generation or two ago, the operation was commonplace. But doctors today feel that such surgery is needed only in extreme cases, such as recurring abcesses.

Are there alternatives to surgery?

Though the drastic drop in operations over the past several decades undoubtedly has spared many children unnecessary surgery, some children who should have had their tonsils removed didn't. Those youngsters are now adults, and they are suffering from chronic sore throats. This problem has triggered research into remedial alternatives to surgery.

One such procedure, developed by Somnus Medical Technologies and ArthroCare, both of Sunnyside, California, involves using radio-frequency technology to shrink the tonsils. The patient gets local anesthesia and sits in a chair as if at a dentist's, opening wide while the doctor inserts a needlelike device that thrusts bursts of heat into each tonsil. The procedure lasts no more than half an hour.

Recovery time is minimal, with most patients returning to work within twenty-four to forty-eight hours.

While studies show that the procedure yields an average 70 percent reduction in tonsil size, some physicians are concerned that it does not truly address the problem—the propensity of the tonsil to become reinfected. Others worry that general anesthesia is not administered. They point out that tonsillectomies are delicate operations, since the tonsils are within two centimeters of the carotid artery (which carries blood to the brain), and that the patient should be immobilized.

Stroke

Strokes, which mostly affect men over sixty, are the third leading cause of death in the United States, trailing only heart disease and cancer. Victims generally have high blood pressure and high cholesterol counts.

What do we mean when we say someone has had a stroke?

We mean that the blood supply to the brain, conveyed by the carotid and vertebral arteries, has been suddenly and drastically interrupted, impairing coordination, sensation, speech, thinking, and vision.

Are there warning signs?

Full-fledged strokes may be preceded by so-called transient ischemic attacks (TIAs), temporary blockages of the blood supply, with minimal damage to the brain.

What are the main kinds of stroke?

Ischemic attacks are those in which either a clot or atherosclerosis blocks the blood vessel, and they are mostly survived. Hemorrhagic attacks are those in which the vessel itself bursts, inducing bleeding in the brain, and are mostly fatal.

Why do strokes affect only one side of the body?

They damage, at any given time, only one of the brain's two hemispheres—either the left or the right.

Since the nerves leading to the brain cross over at the neck, stroke symptoms appear on the opposite side of the body from the impaired hemisphere.

How are strokes diagnosed?

People who have transient ischemic attacks are the most fortunate victims, in the sense that doctors have more time to evaluate their condition.

Speedy diagnoses are all-important, and the most effective tools in this regard are computerized tomography (CT) and magnetic resonance imaging (MRI) scans.

What therapies are there?

Ischemic stroke victims are immediately hospitalized and given anti-coagulants. When their condition improves, they are advised how proper diet and exercise can help their problem. In certain cases, remedial surgery may be performed.

Most people suffering hemorrhagic strokes require emergency surgery. Later, when their condition permits, they likewise are urged to make changes to their lifestyle.

What role does aspirin play in treating ischemic strokes?

Researchers have found that even a few weeks' use of aspirin within forty-eight hours of a stroke decreased the rate of recurrent strokes by a third.

More powerful clot-busting drugs are more effective than aspirin, of course, but they must be given within three to six hours of the attack.

Even in the case of hemorrhagic strokes, where doctors have previously hesitated to give aspirin because it thins the blood, the danger now seems to have been overstated.

Somebody told me that snake venom is being used to treat stroke victims. Is this true?

You were probably being told about ancrod, a substance derived from Malaysian pit vipers. Researchers at the University of Texas Health Center in San Antonio have reported that 42 percent of stroke patients receiving ancrod regained "favorable functional status," compared with 34 percent of patients receiving placebos, and that few patients receiving the venom were left severely disabled.

Ancrod is not likely, however, to replace standard drug therapy for strokes, which is known as tPA and is far easier to administer. The more promising scenario is that the venom will be used in conjunction with tPA and other drugs.

Is stroke a painful syndrome?

Some strokes have associated pain—thalamic pain and shoulder/hand syndrome. Thalamic pain is found in certain localized cerebral lesions and may be intense in nature. Medication and neurological evaluation are usually required.

What is shoulder/hand syndrome?

Shoulder/hand syndrome is a pain syndrome associated with some strokes. The shoulder/hand of the affected limb can present with intense pain, limited range of motion, and change in temperature and coloration. Careful evaluation combined with options of splinting, positioning, mobilization, and medication may be effective.

Do stroke survivors ever make full recoveries?

Some do, but most have to expect some degree of continued impairment.

Much depends, of course, on the survivor's age and positive mental outlook, as well as the quality of the rehabilitative care he or she receives. Impairments that persist for six months are probably permanent.

What is new in stroke rehabilitation therapy?

Researchers have achieved good results with a procedure called constraint-induced movement therapy. The rehabilitation involves immobilizing a good arm or leg so that the patient is forced to use the paralyzed limb for various tasks. In this way the brain literally reorganizes its circuitry, helping people regain partial use of paralyzed limbs in two or three weeks even if the stroke occurred a year or more before.

Therapy calls for concentrated rehabilitation lasting at least six hours a day over a two- or three-week period.

The fact that an adult brain can rewire itself after an injury has been shown in animals for decades, but studies at the University of Alabama and the Friedrich Schiller University of Jena in Germany now have extended the case to humans. Researchers at these institutions postulate that the cells of many stroke victims are not dead but in a state of shock. Every time a patient tries to use an impaired limb and fails, the impairment of the stunned cells is reinforced and the brain falls deeper into despair.

By strapping down the good arm or leg, researchers theorize that the impaired limb will be forced into movement and the brain will "unlearn" its sense of helplessness.

Uterine Pain (cancer, fibroids, prolapsed uterus, dysfunctional bleeding)

Who are most at risk for uterine cancer?

Postmenopausal women; those with a pattern of irregular periods; and those suffering from diabetes, high blood pressure, and obesity.

Where precisely does the cancer develop?

In the endometrium, the lining of the uterus, which normally adds tissue layers each month to host any fertilized eggs. (If no fertilization occurs, the extra tissue is discharged during menstruation.)

What are the symptoms?

Abnormal vaginal bleeding and discharges and possibly a distended uterus. A biopsy is taken to confirm the diagnosis.

How is the cancer treated?

Through a complete hysterectomy, removing the cervix, uterus, ovaries, and fallopian tubes. Sometimes the surgery is followed up with radiation therapy.

What are fibroids, and how do I know if I have them?

They're benign tumors in the uterus. Their growth is related to hormone levels, so pregnancy, oral contraceptives, or estrogen replacement contribute to their development.

Key symptoms are abnormal vaginal bleeding and abdominal pain. Ultrasound scans will verify the presence of fibroids.

Will I need surgery?

Hysterectomies are not always necessary. Fibroids grow slowly or not at all, and most shrink after menopause. If your symptoms are manageable and you can stay away from hormone stimulants, you may be better off adopting a wait-and-see approach.

Meanwhile, you should see your doctor at six-month intervals.

What is a prolapsed uterus?

If you have difficulty urinating or moving your bowels, your uterus may have slipped down, or prolapsed, from the lower abdomen to the vaginal area, putting pressure on both the bladder and the rectum.

How does this condition come about?

Generally, as a result of getting older, becoming obese, or having repeated childbirths.

What can I do about it?

That depends on how far down the uterus has slipped. In some instances, pelvic exercises may strengthen the supporting ligaments sufficiently to keep the organ in place. In more severe cases, a vaginal hysterectomy may be needed to remove the uterus entirely.

To avoid surgery, you may prefer being fitted with a pessary, a diaphragm-like device inserted into the vagina to support the uterus. The drawback here is that the pessary must be replaced every few months.

What is dysfunctional uterine bleeding, and when is it most likely to occur?

This is abnormal bleeding that originates in the endometrium. It results from hormonal changes rather than injury and usually strikes just before and after the reproductive years, with a quarter of the cases affecting teenagers and half affecting women over forty.

What causes the problem?

High levels of estrogen, together with low levels of progesterone—the hormone that prepares the uterus for the fertilized egg. The disparity thickens the endometrial tissues to the point that they "shed," or bleed, heavily and irregularly.

How is it treated?

If the thickened endometrium contains abnormal cells, the condition may be precancerous and require a hysterectomy.

If the cells are normal, the bleeding usually responds to carefully monitored doses of estrogen and progesterone, in combinations designed to regulate the menstrual cycle.

Vascular Leg Pain (varicose veins, phlebitis, lymphedema, cramps)

How do these conditions differ?

- Superficial varicose veins are swollen, bulging, bluish veins in the legs and ankles. Just as the arteries have the job of pushing blood away from the heart, veins have the task of returning it. They accomplish this by a series of one-way valves, which open and close in tandem to move the blood and prevent backflow. If the vein walls weaken, however, the vein widens and the valves don't close properly. The blood engorges, and the result is varicosity.

- Superficial phlebitis is an inflammation of the veins, causing them to harden and redden.

- Lymphedema is swelling in the limbs caused by damage to the lymphatic vessels, which are much smaller than veins and carry nutrients to the tissues.

- Night cramps are painful muscle contractions. Vascular flow, as well as potassium balance in the bloodstream, may be factors in this syndrome.

How are they treated?

- Mild varicose-vein cases benefit from support stockings, elevation of the legs, and the occasional aspirin. More painful conditions require sclerotherapy or even surgery. In sclerotherapy, an outpatient procedure, a solution is injected into the varicose veins to collapse their walls. The blood then finds other, healthier vein paths to return to the heart, and the swollen veins shrink. Surgery calls for removing the longest superficial, or saphenous, vein, which runs from the groin to the ankle, as well as related varicosities. This procedure, called stripping, removes the maximum number of damaged veins at one time. Again, the blood flows upward along healthier pathways.

- Phlebitis usually heals itself, in a week to ten days, with no more help than aspirin.

- Lymphedema patients need to wear support stockings all their waking hours.

- Cramp sufferers should do stretching exercises. Here is one: Lie flat on your back on the floor, feet touching, arms straight over your head, hands touching. Simultaneously flex your ankles and stretch your arms. Hold that position for several seconds, then relax. You will feel muscles tensing, then loosening, the length of your body, from calves to abdomen, from shoulders to arms. Do ten repetitions, building up to twenty-five.

You mention "superficial" varicose veins and phlebitis. Are there other kinds?

Yes, "deep" varicose veins and phlebitis, whose symptoms are extremely difficult to detect, pose life-threatening problems. Both are conditions that lend themselves to blood clots in the vein walls. If the clots break away and travel to the lungs, they can be fatal.

If your pain significantly worsens or the swelling spreads from the vein to the entire leg, see your doctor immediately.

Why does edema hurt?

Edema is harmful fluid accumulation that not only limits mobility but encourages the toxic buildup that irritates the venous system, causing pain.

Because the veins are a low-pressure conduit, the effect of gravity on them is all-important. When someone with varicosity is inactive or standing, the damaged veins find it difficult, if not impossible, to return the blood to the heart. Venous return is compromised, as the medical jargon goes, and edema results.

Elevating the legs and muscle-flexing exercises stimulate "venous return," reducing toxic accrual and the ensuing edema.

A cautionary note: Edema can also be caused by cardiac and kidney problems. This possibility should not be ignored.

What substances that we take into our bodies exacerbate leg pain?

The biggest one by far is cigarette smoke, which causes immediate constriction of the blood supply, as well as long-term vascular problems.

Other substances can be injurious depending on what other illness the vascular sufferer has. Diabetics who ingest sugar, for instance, complicate not only their underlying condition but also their leg pain.

How do the therapies differ for vascular and neurogenic conditions?

Vascular leg pain is relieved by exercise and muscle-flexing, neurogenic pain by rest.

What does the term *claudication* mean?

It's used to describe cramping in the leg, from the Latin word meaning "to limp."

Is age a factor in leg pain?

Vascular problems are more common in older people and may be due to underlying diseases or the long-term intake of toxins.

I'm in my sixties and often feel leg pain while walking. Is this a normal part of the aging process or a sign of incipient vascular disease?

Leg pain in older people can be a sign of what is called peripheral vascular disease, which is caused by blockages in the leg arteries that increase the risk of heart disease. An organization called Legs for Life is cooperating with health-care centers nationwide to offer screenings for the problem.

The procedure begins with a questionnaire that assesses the patient's risk factor—focusing on smoking habits, high cholesterol or blood pressure, being over fifty, or history of heart disease or diabetes. Then the patient undergoes a painless ankle-brachial exam in which ultrasound is used to measure the blood pressure in the ankle and arm. Low blood pressure in the ankle is a sign of blockage in a leg artery.

Treatment for peripheral vascular disease includes cholesterol or blood pressure medication or, as a last resort, surgery on the arteries.

What are leg ulcers?

They are open sores, slow to heal, that develop as a result of vascular disease. The poorer the blood supply, the worse the problem. In extreme cases, they may lead to gangrene and amputation.

Withdrawal—Drug and Alcohol

What is detoxification?

Detox is the medically supervised, physiological process of cleansing the body of toxic substances; it involves the vascular system, liver, kidneys, and even the skin. The process is the first step in helping individuals recover from addiction to narcotics, barbiturates, alcohol, and cigarettes. Detox's most severe withdrawal effects come within the first twenty-four hours, and the full purging takes about two weeks.

Should drug and alcohol problems be treated differently?

Some experts treat the addictions separately, perhaps because of minor differences in withdrawal patterns, related behavior, and relapse rate. But the conditions are essentially the same:

Both involve disrupting one's life with voluntarily taken substances, putting at risk one's mental state, health, career, and personal relationships.

Both involve using these substances to escape physical or emotional pain, ignoring the irony that ever increasing dosages bring only higher tolerance and less relief.

Once the addict understands that (1) his or her actions are voluntary, and therefore can be changed, and (2) in the long run drugs and alcohol are heightening his or her pain, he or she is moving toward recovery.

We feel the two addictions should be treated similarly.

But I only smoke cigarettes. Am I an addict?

Most experts agree that nicotine is a highly addictive substance. With-drawal symptoms are severe, and the relapse rate is higher than for drug or alcohol dependency.

The same experts point out that nicotine is a leading cause of lung cancer, heart disease, and vascular disorders.

In view of these indisputable facts, why do *you* think you con-tinue to smoke? Could it be that you're addicted?

Are the bad effects of heavy drinking accentuated by smoking?

Scientists have long known that tobacco produces adverse changes in the tumor-suppression gene called p53, resulting in an added likeli-hood of lung cancer. Heavy use of alcohol, on the other hand, pre-viously had not been tied to p53 damage.

Now new studies indicate that heavy drinkers who smoke are twice as prone to have p53 damage as nondrinkers who smoke, and five times more likely as those who neither drink nor smoke.

What is behavioral addiction?

It's a dependency on prescription drugs. Barbiturates and benzodiaz-epines, for instance, are commonly prescribed to induce sleep or re-duce anxiety. But if they are taken for too long or at too high a dosage, the patient becomes habituated. Giving up the drugs is difficult, with the attendant withdrawal symptoms.

When I take pain medicine, why do I watch the clock?

Watching the clock may be a warning sign that you are becoming addicted. The permissible time interval between doses, rather than the pain level, is becoming all-important.

You are anticipating pain rather than experiencing it. You are creating your own torment.

When I am withdrawing from a harmful substance, why do I feel so much worse?

Withdrawal symptoms are painful, frightening, and anxiety-provoking. Even while the toxic substance is exiting your body, the craving continues.

Riding through the detox cycle, with appropriate clinical and emotional support, is crucial to recovery. Expect some level of pain during the process. Dealing with it is the price of escaping addiction.

Can acupuncture help in withdrawing from drugs?

A recent study in the *Archives of Internal Medicine* reported that acupuncture helped some cocaine addicts. Half the subjects tested responded favorably to the treatment, while only a quarter responded to "sham" acupuncture procedures.

The study focused on people addicted to both heroin and cocaine. They were receiving methadone for heroin abuse but were still regularly using cocaine. "These are a difficult group of people to deal with," said Dr. Herbert D. Kleber, medical director of the National Center on Addiction and Substance Abuse in New York City, commenting on the findings. "We don't have medicine for treating cocaine addiction, and acupuncture appears to be a useful adjunct for decreasing dependence."

In the treatments, needles were inserted five times a week for about forty-five minutes per session. Dr. Arthur Margolin, a research scientist in the Department of Psychiatry at the Yale Medical School, was the lead author of the report. He theorized that the acupuncture procedure, which is thought to release opioids, the body's natural painkillers, might simultaneously reduce the body's craving for cocaine.

What is recidivism?

It's relapsing into the use of the original drug or substance, as well as the disruptive behavior associated with it.

Denial, anger, and low self-esteem are all part of the addictive profile. This negative behavior tends to re-create itself, making the person more likely to relapse.

While a support network is important in preventing recidivism, it must be composed of people who will not tolerate self-destructive conduct. *Tough love* is the term used to describe this attitude.

Does the twelve-step program work for everybody?

This program, pioneered by Alcoholics Anonymous, emphasizes group meetings, peer pressure, and a quasi-evangelical atmosphere. Over the years it has been used to combat not only alcoholism but many forms of addiction. It is a very positive and easy-to-understand program and can be applied to people with a broad range of cultural and educational backgrounds.

That said, it's important to remember that the twelve-step program has never claimed a 100 percent success rate and was never meant to treat all disorders. Many people may be more comfortable with more sophisticated therapy specifically designed for the individual and administered by professional clinicians.

Pain Postscript

by Mathew H. M. Lee, M.D.

We know that great strides are now being made in the area of pain management. How would you sum up these developments?

Do you remember when you were a child and you fell and hurt yourself, and your mom was always there to take care of you? Well, now that you're an adult, you should expect pain experts to give you the same level of comfort. MOM is the three-letter acronym I've created for this kind of compassionate care: *m* for measurement, *o* for open-mindedness, *m* for meditation.

What do you mean by "measurement"?

You'll recall that we encourage patients to keep a written account of the pain they feel each day, as well as when they feel it and how it waxes and wanes. This helps them come to grips with the causal factors that are influencing their discomfort and helps the doctors in prescribing treatment.

But now the new weapon we have in pain measurement is the emerging science of thermography, which enables us to create photographs that pinpoint the pain and the degree to which it is being felt. Such diagnoses are a cornerstone of the approach we take at the Rusk Institute.

How does thermography work?

Each person has a distinct skin-surface temperature pattern. Pain causes a reduction in circulation, which makes certain areas cooler. These changes reflect physical reactions, which may be normal—like the chill in your hands on a wintry day—or may be abnormal, the result of some trauma or disease.

In clinical thermography the patient's skin temperatures are visualized through some thirty infrared images, from hot red to cool blue. A damaged left knee, for instance, would show up in blue and green hues while the undamaged knee in the other leg would be in red and purple.

Thermography enables us to search for pain. Once we find it, we can do something about it.

What do you mean by "open-mindedness"?

In part, I mean that the medical profession has for too long been close-minded, or even uncaring, in the treatment of pain. Some doctors have even said, in effect, Grin and bear the discomfort. During the 1990s a study in the *New England Journal of Medicine* found that 42 percent of cancer outpatients were not given adequate pain relievers; during the same decade the U.S. Department of Health stated that 50 percent of surgical patients received insufficient postop medication.

Fortunately, that attitude is fast disappearing. Just last year the Joint Commission on Accreditation of Healthcare Organizations, which supervises most of the country's medical facilities, ordered new criteria for identifying and treating pain. Now doctors and nurses—in the drug field, for instance—have to educate themselves about new medications and how they interrelate to one another.

In the larger picture, the Joint Commission's mandates mean that courses on pain management will become part of the basic curriculum at medical schools and hospitals. Sufferers clearly will benefit.

How else can the medical community show its open-mindedness?

By accepting the possibility that alternative treatments can in some cases be as effective as conventional ones, or at least be helpful supplements. Don't misunderstand me. The conventional treatments for cancer, for instance, are chemotherapy, radiation, and surgery, and I would be the last person to suggest that a cancer patient not avail himself or herself of these procedures if necessary. But in the area of pain management, there are often many different ways to treat people.

One of my own subspecialties is acupuncture, which I have been using for decades and about which many people have misinformed ideas. Most acupuncturists in the United States today are not medical doctors and know little of modern neurophysiology. They follow the classical Asian approach, which involves identifying 365 points of stimulation, a number so large that its practice obviously lends itself to varying degrees of hocus-pocus.

Physicians like me use acupuncture not to replace traditional care but to supplement what we know with certainty about neurophysiology. We see the procedure as a stimulant for the central nervous system—releasing endorphins that help relieve pain. It's a big medical world out there. Let's take advantage of it.

When you mention the big world out there, one thinks of the Internet. What do you think of the fact that more and more people are getting their medical information from the Net?

This phenomenon is like anything else: its effectiveness lies in how the data are utilized. Open-mindedness again is the keyword. Physicians should realize that informed patients are the best kind of patients. The very fact that sick people are taking the trouble to do research means they *want* to lead healthy lives. Doctors should be appreciative of this effort.

Conversely, patients should appreciate that a little knowledge can be dangerous. Don't treat yourself. Take your findings to your physician and discuss them. In many instances the reports on the Net are experimental and may do more harm than good.

For the terminally ill, of course, even clinical trials can offer much-needed hope, and in this regard the Net can be a godsend. The fact that a couple of hundred people have generally benefited from an experimental procedure or drug can be enormously encouraging to someone who has a similar illness, warding off depression. The National Library of Medicine's ClinicalTrials.gov Web site, launched only last year, has data on more than 5,200 trials, mostly those sponsored by the National Institutes of Health.

What about the third letter in the acronym? What do you mean when you call for "meditation"?

By this I mean that everyone in the pain-management field should realize that the calming influence of the mind—through meditation, prayer, interaction with the Godhead, however you want to describe spirituality—can with proper training to some degree offset the ravages of the body.

How this happens I don't know, but I have seen the phenomenon in my patients again and again. I can only speculate that meditation stimulates the production of T cells, those white blood cells that mature in the thymus and play various roles in strengthening the immune system and rejecting foreign agents.

Certainly meditation leads to optimism, and many studies have shown that optimists create less stress and fewer mood disturbances for themselves and are more likely to exercise and to eat and drink in moderation. If you use your mind to help your body, you will be the better for it.

Measurement, open-mindedness, meditation—these are the tools we use at the Rusk Institute to supplement traditional medicine. All across the country, I am happy to say, more and more pain clinics are following similar procedures, showing patients how to cope with pain.